MANAGING PAIN

And Other Medically Proven
Uses of Acupuncture

Dr Richard Halvorsen

First edition published by Gibson Square

info@gibsonsquare.com
www.gibsonsquare.com
Tel: +44 (0)20 7096 1100 (UK)
Tel: +1 646 216 9813 (USA)
Tel: +353 (0)1 657 1057 (Eire)

ISBN   9781908096852

Printed and bound by CPI Group (UK) Ltd, Croydon, CR0 4YY

Contents

Introduction 5

Frequently Asked Questions

1 What Is Acupuncture? 13
2 What Are the Treatments? 21
3 What Happens during Treatment? 27
4 Is Acupuncture Safe? 31
5 What Can Acupuncture Treat? 37

Managing Pain and Treating Diseases

6 Musculoskeletal Problems 40
7 Headaches & Migraines 54
8 Female (Gynaecological) Problems 60
9 Conditions Related to Pregnancy 74
10 Asthma and Allergic Conditions 82
11 Addictions 88
12 Bowel Problems 94
13 Psychological Problems 100

14 Cancer   106

15 Other Conditions   112

16 What Is Acupuncture Unable to Treat?   137

Appendices

I   How Do I Find a Good Acupuncturist?   141

II Research into Acupuncture   151

III Resources (UK, Australia, New Zealand)   156

Index   160

Introduction

When I was training to be a doctor in London in the 1980s we were not taught anything about acupuncture. There was no mention of it during my five years of study, except possibly the odd aside by a consultant who mocked a patient for being so silly as to seek some acupuncture before coming round to their senses and seeing a 'proper doctor'. We were not informed about any of the so-called 'complementary' or 'alternative' therapies. Acupuncture, along with all the others, was considered unscientific and mysterious – and not something with which serious doctors should be dabbling.

However, as a medical student, and then a junior hospital doctor, I frequently and repeatedly saw patients suffering from chronic medical conditions for whom our 'proper' scientific medicine had little to offer.

Western medicine did not have all the answers, and I wondered whether other systems of medicine might be able to fill in some of the gaps. Soon after finishing my medical studies I embarked on a two year course in Traditional Chinese Acupuncture at the British College of Acupuncture (which sadly no longer exists) in London.

Traditional Chinese Medicine (TCM) is based on a completely different system of medicine from the one I had been taught in medical school. I started by trying to relate what I was being taught to what I had learnt at medical school. In TCM there is talk of the kidney, the liver and the heart; at least I knew, or thought I knew, what these were. I assumed a kidney was the same kidney and a liver was the same liver in any system.

Wrong. In modern medicine the kidneys are seen as organs that filter the blood, preserving the chemical balance of the blood and producing urine. In TCM the kidneys are believed to store the body's 'Essence'; amongst other functions they produce marrow and manufacture blood. This is complete nonsense to a Western trained doctor and so six months into my course I was feeling totally confused. Then the penny dropped. I would no longer think of a TCM kidney as being the same thing as a Western medical kidney. I realized that they were completely different concepts, similar only in that they share a common name.

I no longer believed literally what I was being taught (I knew that the kidneys didn't really manufacture blood) but saw this way of explaining the body as a template on which to devise a traditional Chinese treatment. The important thing to me, as a clinician, was whether the treatment worked; I was less concerned about the theoretical foundation on which that treatment was based.

During, and after, my course I was able to see acupuncture being used in practice and saw with my own eyes that it often, though not always, did work and sometimes even relieved people from distressing symptoms that orthodox Western medicine, the one I had studied in medical school, hadn't been able to help.

In subsequent years I continued to study both traditional Chinese and Western medical acupuncture in the UK and China. I have also received acupuncture myself for various problems over the years.

A lot has changed during my time in practice over the last 30 years. In the early years my practice of acupuncture was received, at best, with baffled amusement and, at worst, with strong condemnation. Now thousands of doctors have received training in acupuncture and many use it as part of their daily practice. I receive frequent referrals from both consultants and GPs, something that did not happen not too long ago. Acupuncture is increasingly used by GPs themselves, or provided by other members of the primary health care team, such as physiotherapists or nurses.

8 *Dr Richard Halvorsen*

Acupuncture is now one of the most popular of all complementary therapies. Over one million people in Great Britain and nearly two million Australians (over nine per cent of the adult population) use acupuncture every year. Nearly twenty million people in the USA have used acupuncture at one time or another. Though it is still not easy for most people to obtain acupuncture treatment on the NHS, it is widely available privately. But finding an experienced and competent acupuncturist is a minefield as anyone, even with little or no training or qualifications, can legally call themselves an 'acupuncturist'.

I set out to make this the first book that looks at acupuncture from both a Western and Chinese perspective, rather than favouring just one of them. I seek to explain our understanding of how acupuncture works, both from a traditional Chinese viewpoint and from a modern Western scientific perspective.

I have also pulled together all the up-to-date medical evidence and merged this with my extensive clinical experience to give the most comprehensive, yet easy to use, guide to what acupuncture can effectively treat. I find that most acupuncture resources either make claims that acupuncture can treat virtually everything (clearly not the case) or, by applying an overzealous scientific approach, conclude that acupuncture is no more than a placebo (again not so and contradicting much research).

By amalgamating the science with clinical experience I believe this book is the first to bridge the divide between Western and Chinese approaches to acupuncture to provide a balanced overview of the benefits of acupuncture. This book is, in particular, aimed at those with little or no knowledge of acupuncture and to assist those who may be thinking of seeking acupuncture treatment, but will hopefully also be of use to the practitioners of either perspective.

There has been an increasing amount of research into acupuncture over recent decades and we are now beginning to understand how it works and the many ways it can affect the body – from a scientific perspective. More importantly, from a practical standpoint, we are learning which conditions are most likely to be helped by acupuncture and which problems would be better treated with other approaches. Research, and scientific evidence, is extremely important but this needs to be used alongside clinical experience. I have been using acupuncture to treat my patients for over a quarter of a century and have seen what it can – and can't – do with my own eyes. I never cease to be amazed when people, who have already been to see several specialists without benefit, are quite quickly and dramatically helped by acupuncture. Of course acupuncture is not a miracle cure and not everyone, or all conditions, can be successfully treated with acupuncture.

Many common conditions will be examined and how likely it is that these can be successfully treated with acupuncture. You may be nervous at the thought of having needles put in you, but most people do not find this particularly uncomfortable. Below you'll find out what you can expect to happen when you visit an acupuncturist and also the (very occasional) things that can go wrong.

Frequently Asked Questions

1

What Is Acupuncture?

Acupuncture is a treatment that involves inserting extremely fine needles into the skin. It has been used in China for over two thousand years, and has increasingly been used in the West since the 1970s.

It is used to relieve symptoms of, and sometimes help cure, a variety of physical and psychological conditions and may encourage the body's ability to heal itself.

Over the past thirty years there has been considerable scientific research into acupuncture and we are now beginning to understand how it works. We can be confident that the effects of acupuncture are not all in the mind.

The distinction between complementary, or alternative, medicine and orthodox medicine is becoming blurred as the benefits of acupuncture become accepted by conventional doctors. It is increasingly being used alongside conventional medicine, is used in the vast majority of NHS pain clinics and is being offered by an ever increasing number of GPs and hospital doctors.

There are several variations on the traditional method in which fine needles are inserted into the skin in the appropriate parts of the body. For example, there is auriculotherapy (or ear acupuncture) in which needles are only inserted into the ears, and electro-acupuncture in which the acupuncture needles are stimulated with an electric current. (*These are described in chapter 2.*)

There are two fundamentally different approaches to acupuncture. It is important to understand these as most acupuncturists will use exclusively, or predominantly, one or other system.

Acupuncture as part of Traditional Chinese Medicine

Traditional Chinese acupuncture is based on traditional Chinese medicine (TCM), an ancient system of medicine originating in the East two thousand years ago.

This is based on the belief that energy (or Qi, pronounced 'chee') flows throughout the body along channels or 'meridians'. Balance and harmony are integral to the concept of health and any obstruction to the smooth flow of Qi throughout the body can cause disease. The concept of harmony is also represented in the balance between Yin and Yang. The principle that everyone is governed by the opposing, but complementary, forces of Yin and Yang is central to Chinese philosophy.

It is believed that pain, or illness, occurs if the body becomes out of balance and the energy (Qi) is prevented from flowing freely. The purpose of acupuncture is to remove any blockages and enable the energy to flow freely and harmoniously throughout the body, thereby restoring balance and health.

Practitioners also believe that acupuncture can be used as preventive medicine to help maintain, or improve, a person's wellbeing, a concept that is alien to a practitioner of Western medical acupuncture (see below).

TCM traditionally includes the use of other treatment modalities alongside acupuncture. These include the administration of Chinese herbs, a type of massage or manipulative therapy called 'Tui na' and a form of exercise (qi gong, pronounced 'chee gong') which balances breathing, movement and awareness.

The TCM acupuncturist will not make a Western diagnosis but a TCM diagnosis and treat the patient accordingly.

For example, a 35 year old man may suffer from pain in the upper abdomen (pit of the stomach), chest discomfort and belching. A Western diagnosis might be gastritis (inflammation of the stomach), whereas a TCM diagnosis could be 'an attack of the stomach by hyperactive liver Qi'. This TCM diagnosis, though meaningless to a Western trained doctor, will enable a TCM trained practitioner to insert acupuncture needles in appropriate points along the correct meridians in order to disperse the liver Qi and regulate the stomach Qi.

To take one further example, nettle rash or urticaria is a common skin condition that is generally believed in Western medicine to be allergic in origin even though, more often then not, the allergic cause cannot be found. However, a TCM practitioner may diagnose this as 'pathogenic wind in the muscles', completely nonsensical to a Western trained doctor but again informing the Chinese acupuncturist where to put the needles.

It is not only as if the two systems of medicine have different languages, but languages that cannot even be translated into each other.

Western Medical Acupuncture

Western scientific acupuncture does not accept the existence of meridians and rejects the traditional Chinese philosophy on which this is based. Practitioners argue that acupuncture works by stimulating the nervous system through which the body's organs can be affected and hormones released.

Western Medical Acupuncture builds on the traditional knowledge and immense experience of the Chinese by adapting it using our current knowledge of anatomy, along with the principles of evidence based medicine. Less importance is placed on the traditional concepts of Qi, Yin and Yang. Instead, acupuncture is seen to act primarily by stimulating the nervous system and by its ability to stimulate the release of a wide variety of chemicals and hormones in the body.

Though traditional acupuncture points are commonly used, points are also selected because they are trigger points, or because they connect to the part of the body being treated via the spinal cord (segmental acupuncture).

There are five mechanisms by which acupuncture is known to work:

1. Local stimulation

Acupuncture needles stimulate nerve endings in the skin and muscle where the needles are inserted. This causes the release of various substances and an increase in blood flow (which can often be seen as a redness in the skin surrounding the needle) all of which encourage healing.

2. Segmental acupuncture

The needles stimulate the level, or 'segment', of the

spinal cord that connects – via nerves – with the area of skin or muscle that the needle is inserted in. This helps relieve pain in the affected area, but can also have an effect, in ways that we do not yet fully understand, on the internal organs of the body that are also connected to the same level of the spinal cord.

3. Extrasegmental acupuncture

The insertion of the needle stimulates not only the segment into which it is inserted but this stimulation then travels up the spinal cord to the lowest part of the brain (the brainstem) where the body's own pain controlling mechanisms are stimulated into action. This effect is similar to what happens when, for example, you injure yourself playing sport and you don't really notice it until afterwards when it then hurts more. During the game the body's own pain suppressing mechanisms (which can be stimulated by acupuncture) were in action.

4. Central regulatory effects

Acupuncture has an effect on many parts of the brain, and this has been demonstrated in brain scans. It has a calming effect on many patients and improves their wellbeing. It influences various hormones such as the female hormones controlling the menstrual cycle and fertility.

5. Trigger point acupuncture

Trigger points are tight knots of muscle that can be extremely painful especially when pressed. They arise out of injury, either a sudden accident (a whiplash injury is a classic cause of trigger points in the muscles of the neck, though they can form from something as simple as lifting something too heavy) or long-term overuse (trigger points are usually found in the muscles of a repetitive strain injury or RSI).

In reality we are a long way from understanding fully how acupuncture works scientifically. However, research, though poorly funded (it is of no interest to the big pharmaceutical companies who fund the majority of medical research), is enlightening us more all the time about how acupuncture works. In addition real-time scans of the brain are beginning to show how acupuncture exerts effects on deeper structures within the brain.

Most acupuncturists will practice either TCM acupuncture or Western medical acupuncture, though a few who have been trained in both methods will use a synthesis of the two systems or will pick whichever is most appropriate for the problem in front of them. Over the years there has been some friction between practitioners of TCM acupuncture, most of whom do not have a medical or paramedical training, and the doctors and other health professionals who practice Western medical acupuncture. The TCM acupuncturists, or 'professional acupuncturists' as they prefer to be called have mainly undergone extensive training of at least three years in TCM. They resent the fact that some doctors will start practicing a simplified form of acupuncture after only a couple of weekends training. On the other hand, doctors and other health professionals voice their concerns that 'lay acupuncturists' without formal medical training should not be practicing acupuncture in the absence of medical supervision as they might miss important diagnoses that should be treated with orthodox medicine. I'm relieved to say that over recent years this acrimony has abated somewhat and the two groups, though still functioning independently, now share a wary respect for each other. In practice there is a significant overlap in the two types of treatment. Doctors will frequently use the more common 'big' traditional acupuncture points, and TCM acupuncturists will use what the Chinese call 'Ah Shi' or 'ouch' points which often correspond to trigger points.

2

What Are the Treatments?

Needles

Most acupuncture treatments will simply involve inserting extremely fine needles in various parts of the body.
These may be stimulated, to a greater or lesser degree,
by hand. This is by far the most common form of
acupuncture.

Electro-acupuncture

Sometimes, pairs of acupuncture needles are attached
via leads to a machine that generates mild electrical
pulses. This provides an extra stimulation that can be
useful in some conditions that are difficult to treat and
require a more powerful 'dose' of acupuncture, such as
painful conditions that are not responding to regular
acupuncture.

Electro-acupuncture may be felt by the patient as a
tingling sensation and may also sometimes cause

muscles to twitch where the needles are inserted. Electro-acupuncture is also used in specific conditions like stroke and addictions. There are occasional situations in which electro-acupuncture should not be used, for example across the chest in someone with a cardiac pacemaker.

Moxibustion

Moxibustion is a traditional Chinese practice in which a herb, mugwort or 'Moxa', is attached to the handle of the acupuncture needle and slowly burnt. This creates a warm feeling where the needle is inserted, which is believed to expel cold and warm the meridians leading to the smoother flow of blood and Qi. As the moxa actually burns there is a danger of this falling onto, and burning, the skin. The moxa is sometimes placed directly on the skin and set alight and then removed before it can burn the skin. In traditional practice the burning moxa is occasionally left to burn the skin resulting in a scar, though this is rarely done in the West. The risk of burning to the skin is reduced by using a moxa stick which is held over the acu-point, a treatment that does not require the insertion of needles.

Trigger Point Acupuncture

This type of acupuncture is very popular with doctors

and physiotherapists using a Western form of acupuncture. Many painful muscular conditions, such as neck pain, headaches, tennis elbow and low back pain, result from painful knots of muscle called trigger points. These may have been caused by an injury or simply by longstanding mis- or over-use. This can be an uncomfortable treatment, but is often very successful in relieving the pain and tension associated with the presence of the trigger points. Pain relief is achieved by needling directly into the trigger point, thereby deactivating it and enabling the immediate release of the tight band of muscle. Needling trigger points is often accompanied by twitches of the muscle being needled, which some find disconcerting but most are reassured when told that each twitch is associated with the disappearance of a painful trigger point.

Ear (auricular) acupuncture

Ear acupuncture is based on the belief that the whole body, including all the internal organs, is represented on the ear. In the same way that a reflexologist believes that he or she is able to reach the whole of the body through the foot, so the auricular acupuncturist believes that the ear is the gateway to the whole body, external and internal. Very small needles are inserted into the external ear during the treatment;

some practitioners send patients away with indwelling needles left in the ear covered with a plaster to keep them in place. This is not advisable as there is a small risk of infection which can be serious. A safer alternative is to stick metal balls over the ear acu-points and ask the patient to intermittently rub these to provide stimulation to the points.

Ear acupuncture is commonly used to treat addictions (such as smoking and drug addiction) though its advocates recommend its use for a wide variety of conditions.

Laser acupuncture

Laser acupuncture uses a very fine beam of light, instead of a needle, to stimulate the acu-point. The main advantage of this type of acupuncture is that no needles are involved and so it is completely painless. There is some evidence for its effectiveness but many acupuncturists see it as a milder form of treatment than 'needle' acupuncture. It is a useful alternative for those who are intolerant of needling.

Acupressure

Another needle-free, but not necessarily pain-free, variation of acupuncture is acupressure. The practitioner will press over selected acu-points, a little like having a massage, instead of inserting needles.

Cupping

Cupping is not strictly related to acupuncture but is an ancient therapeutic method that is sometimes used by acupuncturists practicing traditional Chinese acupuncture. The air inside a glass cup is heated and the rim of the cup placed over the skin, typically on the back. As the air in the cup cools it creates a partial vacuum causing the cup to stick to the skin, which is sucked up a little way into the cup. This causes an increase in blood flow to the area; it is used in traditional Chinese medicine to improve the flow of Qi, and thereby treat various conditions.

Cosmetic acupuncture

Cosmetic acupuncture has become increasingly popular over recent years in our, ultimately futile, yearning to stay young, or at least young looking, for as long as possible. Needles are placed in the face and elsewhere on the body to, it is claimed, combat the signs of ageing and to treat skin disorders. Many of the claims for what has been described as an 'acupuncture face-lift' are unsustainable (*See chapter 15*).

3

What Happens during
Treatment?

History

An acupuncture consultation and treatment may be quite unlike anything you have experienced before. However, it is likely to start off in a similar way to any visit to a doctor or other health professional. You will be asked about your problem and why you are considering acupuncture. The acupuncturist will ask you questions about your complaint and your previous medical history. You may be asked questions that appear unrelated to your condition, especially if you visit an acupuncturist practicing traditional Chinese acupuncture (TCM); you may be asked about your sleeping pattern, appetite, digestion, and emotional wellbeing.

Examination (including tongue and pulses if TCM)

A TCM acupuncturist will feel your pulses in both

your wrists where 12 different pulses (six in each wrist) corresponding to the 12 primary meridians can be felt. You may also be asked to stick out your tongue, though both these examinations are likely to be omitted by an acupuncturist practicing Western acupuncture.

Before lying down on a couch you are likely to be asked to roll up your sleeves and take off your socks or tights. You may be asked to remove more clothes than you expected as needles are often inserted in places far away from where the problem is. The acupuncturist may feel your abdomen for tenderness and may prod various areas of the body or measure along the skin with his or her fingers looking for particular points to insert the needles.

Treatment

Then comes the time for insertion of the needles; after all, this is what acupuncture is all about. You will usually be asked to lie down which reduces the (uncommon) risk of feeling faint. Sometimes, however, it may be more appropriate to be treated sitting up on the couch or in a chair. The needles used are extremely fine and may be anything from 15mm to 50mm (or occasionally longer) in length depending on which part of the body they are to be inserted, though most will be around 25 to 30 mm long. They should always be sterile single use disposable needles. Do check this with your acupuncturist; there is no longer any reason to use reusable needles that have to be sterilized between patients.

You should barely feel the needle as it is inserted just under the skin. The needle may then be pushed in a little deeper as the acupuncturist attempts to find the acupuncture point lying beneath the skin, or looks for a muscle trigger point. The acupuncturist will be looking for you to feel a sensation, known as De Qi (pronounced De Chee); you may feel this as a dull ache, a warmth, numbness or tingling.

The sensation may be quite different to anything you have felt before, and everyone feels the needles a little differently, but you will soon get to know the sensation and be able to tell the acupuncturist exactly when he or she has 'hit the spot'. A twitch may be felt, especially in trigger point treatment. The needles may be twiddled a little bit to increase the 'strength' of the treatment, and may also be twiddled again during the treatment. The needles may be left in for 10 to 20 minutes, rarely longer, but may also be removed very soon after treatment in trigger point acupuncture. The needles are usually left alone but may be attached to an electrical stimulator (for electro-acupuncture) or have burning moxa placed on the handles.

You will almost certainly have needles placed around the area where you have the problem, but may also have needles placed in other parts of the body, especially the feet, hands, legs and arms.

The number of needles used varies widely between practitioners. You may be treated with just a single needle (though this is unusual) or have up to 20 (rarely more) needles inserted; 8-15 needles is common.

As you lie with the needles in you probably won't be aware of most of them; though you may have a persistent sensation where they are inserted, which is fine. They should not be unduly painful and if any are you should let the acupuncturist know immediately.

The number of treatments needed varies widely and depends very much on the condition being treated. A simple muscular pain or strain may require only one or two treatments, whereas relief from a long-term condition such as migraine or arthritis may necessitate indefinite treatments, though hopefully at increased intervals as time goes on.

After the treatments you may feel unusually relaxed or even sleepy; with luck you will have a good night's sleep. You may notice an improvement in your symptoms, though this may well take more than one treatment. Sometimes, particularly with painful musculoskeletal conditions there may be a temporary aggravation: the pain may feel a little worse for a day, or two at the most, and when this happens it should normally be followed by an improvement. An aggravation is not necessary, however, for an improvement to occur and most will get better without any worsening of their symptoms.

4

Is Acupuncture Safe?

Acupuncture is extremely safe – provided it is administered by a competent acupuncturist.

In a survey of 66,000 acupuncture treatments published in the British Medical Journal no side-effects were reported that were considered 'serious'.[1,2]

There were a total of 43 events described as 'significant'; these included:

6	occurrences of fainting
5	needles left in patients after treatment
1	skin infection
2	patients who felt anxious or panicked
3	patients who felt sick or vomited

All 43 problems cleared within a week, except for one patient who experienced pain that lasted for two weeks before resolving.

The most serious complication of acupuncture

that I have personally experienced over 25 years of practicing is of one patient who fainted.

Mild side-effects

The most common side-effects experienced by patients receiving acupuncture treatments are:

1   Pain or discomfort on needle insertion
2   Bleeding from the needle site – nearly always very mild and transient
3   Worsening of symptoms – usually temporary and likely to be followed by an improvement. This 'aggravation' is more common in painful conditions and rarely last more than 24-48 hours.

Serious reactions

Serious side-effects, and even deaths, have extremely rarely been reported after acupuncture. The most 'common', or perhaps I should say least rare, side-effect is that of a pneumothorax – or collapsed lung. This is caused by having a needle inserted into the lung cavity and should never occur when being treated by an experienced acupuncturist with good anatomical knowledge. There have only ever been seven deaths recorded anywhere in the world as a result of acupuncture. This may sound alarming but when one considers that billions of acupuncture treatments have been given over many, many years, this is actually very reassuring and makes acupuncture far safer than most other forms of treatment.

Acupuncture has been reported to have caused the transmission of infections such as hepatitis B, but this can only occur if needles are re-used and this risk is the most important reason to use only sterile single-use disposable needles.

Even these can, exceptionally rarely, allow susceptible places like joints to become infected if needled directly.

The main concern of many doctors who practice acupuncture is that important diagnoses could be missed by a non-medically qualified acupuncturist and a patient might be treated with acupuncture when it is more appropriate to have conventional treatment. It has been suggested that this is far less likely to happen if the acupuncturist finds out about your medical history and informs your GP that you are receiving acupuncture. One solution to this is to get a conventional western medical diagnosis first or, failing that, to see your doctor if your condition is not improving with acupuncture. But it only fair at add that there is no evidence that important diagnoses are being missed by TCM acupuncturists or that they are treating people with acupuncture inappropriately.

How does acupuncture compare on safety with other treatments?

This is where acupuncture really scores well as it a good deal safer than many drugs that are used for similar conditions.

Acupuncture is often used in painful conditions for which anti-inflammatory painkillers (NSAIDs) such as Nurofen (ibuprofen) are used. If you bear in mind that these drugs cause over two and a half thousand deaths every year in the UK alone, then this demonstrates how exceptionally safe acupuncture is in competent hands.[3]

Is there anyone who cannot have acupuncture?

There are very few people who cannot have acupuncture.

Clearly great care needs to be taken when putting needles into anyone on anticoagulation (blood thinning) medication such as Warfarin; however there is no reason why gentle acupuncture cannot be given using needles that are not inserted deeply.

Needles should not be inserted in areas of skin that are damaged or infected.

Electro-acupuncture should not be used on someone with a heart pacemaker inserted.

Indwelling needles that remain in the skin outside the treatment room should probably never be used because of the risk of infection, but certainly not in anyone with a deficient immune system or with damaged or artificial heart valves.

Can acupuncture be used in pregnancy?

Traditionally there are certain points that are 'forbidden' for use in pregnancy; however there is no evidence that use of these points is harmful. My view is that acupuncture can be used cautiously in pregnancy, and needles should probably not be inserted into the abdomen especially in the later stages of pregnancy. However, I feel it would be very wrong to withhold acupuncture treatments that are known to help problems that are common in pregnancy, such as early morning sickness and back pain.

1   White A, Hayhoe S, Hart A, Ernst E. Adverse events following acupuncture: prospective survey of 32,000 consultations with doctors and physiotherapists. BMJ 2001; 323: 485-6.

2   MacPherson H, Thomas K, Walters S, Fitter M. The York acupuncture safety study: prospective survey of 34,000 treatments by traditional acupuncturists. BMJ 2001; 323: 486-7.

3   Bandoler. NSAIDs and adverse effects.
http://www.medicine.ox.ac.uk/bandolier/booth/painpag/nsae/nsae.html#Heading11.

5

What Can Acupuncture Treat?

Over recent years there has been a surge of research into acupuncture and whether it can help treat various conditions. Though the amount of research is tiny compared to that done into prescription drugs (which is mainly paid for by the pharmaceutical industry to demonstrate the value of their products), it is nevertheless substantial and increasing all the time.

The following chapters list many of the more common conditions for which acupuncture is used. In each case the likelihood of someone with each condition being helped – based on the scientific research and my clinical experience.

For each condition the following will be discussed:

1 The likelihood of being helped by acupuncture
2 The number and frequency of treatments likely to be needed

3 The evidence supporting acupuncture's effectiveness

4 My own clinical experience

This is inevitably only a guide and the response to acupuncture varies from person to person. Even in conditions for which acupuncture is unlikely to help it may be worth trying if there are no safe and effective alternative treatments.

In addition, each condition has a simplified star-rating of the likelihood of someone being helped by acupuncture:

●●●●●   Most people will be helped by acupuncture

●●●●   There is a good chance that acupuncture will help

●●●   Response is variable, some are definitely helped but others are not

●●   Acupuncture may help some people, but most are unlikely to be helped

○   Acupuncture is unlikely to help

Managing Pain
&
Treating Diseases

6

Musculoskeletal Problems

Low back pain is extremely common, affecting 9 out of every 10 of us at some stage in our lives. Back pain is second only to the common cold as a cause of days lost at work. Acupuncture is widely used to treat low back pain and various trials and reviews have shown that acupuncture is an effective treatment for low back pain.[1,2,3] However, some research suggests that actually having acupuncture needles inserted is more important than where they are put. Not all acupuncturists would agree with this. I, myself, place considerable importance on my patient experiencing a sensation the Chinese call De Qi (pronounced 'De Chee'); this may be felt as a warmth, tingling, dull ache or numbness and is considered by many acupuncturists to be an important guide to the patient's response to acupuncture.

To treat low back pain, needles are usually inserted in the lower back in the region where pain is felt. Some acupuncturists will also insert needles in other points, for example in the arms and legs.

Low back pain usually requires at least 4-6 treatments to get on top of the pain, though longstanding pain may require more treatments.

In 2009 the NICE (the National Institute for Clinical Excellence) recommended that all patients with low back pain should be offered a course of acupuncture, an exercise programme or a course of manual therapy, such as osteopathy.[4] This means that acupuncture should be widely available on the NHS but sadly it isn't. Not many people who go to their GP with back pain and request a course of acupuncture treatment will be able to obtain this on the NHS, despite the NICE recommendation.

Likelihood of being helped by acupuncture ●●●●●

There has been little research on the effect of acupuncture on *neck pain*, a common complaint especially in those who spend many hours a day in front of a computer terminal. In my practice in the City of London I treat many people with neck pain and my experience is that acupuncture usually helps and that most patients appear to get significant pain relief after only a few treatments.

The little research that has been done is encouraging.[5] Neck pain is a condition that is particularly amenable to western 'trigger point' acupuncture rather than traditional Chinese acupuncture.[6]

Acupuncture works at least as well as physiotherapy for chronic neck pain, and possibly slightly better than physiotherapy if pain is particularly bad.[7]

A course of 3-4 treatments involving needling local points in the neck, upper back (from where pain is often 'referred' or transmitted to the neck and surrounding area) is usually sufficient to establish whether acupuncture is likely to help you. You may then need further treatments especially if the cause, such as working in front of a PC, persists; in this case indefinite, but infrequent, 'top-up' treatments of, say, one every three months can be very helpful in keeping the pain at bay.

Likelihood of being helped by acupuncture ●●●●●

Around ten million people in the UK suffer from arthritis. All types of arthritis can cause severe ongoing pain and this can have a profoundly disabling effect on the sufferer. *Osteoarthritis* (often, perhaps incorrectly, referred to as 'wear and tear' arthritis) is by far the most common type of arthritis and is more likely to affect us as we get older.

Though acupuncture is unable to 'cure' arthritis, it can be extremely helpful in relieving the debilitating pain that this condition can cause.

Acupuncture can relive the pain of arthritis in many joints, including the knee, hip, and thumb, though the evidence is particularly strong for osteoarthritis of the knee.[8,9]

Mrs. K, aged 71, first came to see me with a painful thumb that prevented her from picking things up and opening bottles when I was her GP. Her right thumb was affected and as she was right-handed this was even more disabling. We first tried painkillers and anti-inflammatory drugs but these were of little help. I then suggested acupuncture and after four treatments she was completely pain free.

I was delighted and surprised to see her again eight years later in my acupuncture practice after I had left general practice. Her thumb pain had returned and she had tracked me down in my City clinic for some more acupuncture treatments. I gave her two further treatments after which she left pain-free and delighted. I joked that I would see her again in another eight years.

Mrs. K responded particularly well and not everyone is helped so quickly. Between 6 and 12 treatments may be required to get on top of the pain in those who have had the problem for many years. This is often followed by occasional 'top-up' treatments, like with Mrs. K, as acupuncture cannot cure arthritis, but can only relieve the pain of the condition. If ordinary acupuncture is not helping after a few treatments, I may add in electro-acupuncture as this can often work where 'simple' acupuncture is insufficient. Moxibustion may also help relieve the pain of arthritis and other rheumatic conditions.[10]

Though not everyone is helped, acupuncture can be sufficiently effective in relieving the pain of sufferers who had been on the waiting list for joint replacement surgery so that they no longer need the operation.[11]

Likelihood of being helped by acupuncture ●●●●

Rheumatoid arthritis (RA) is an auto-immune disease that causes inflammation of the joints resulting in pain and swelling. It is the second most common form of arthritis in the UK. Women are more commonly affected than men and the disease typically starts in midlife. Orthodox treatments include medication in the form of painkillers, anti-inflammatory drugs, steroids and disease-modifying agents as well as physiotherapy and occasionally surgery. Acupuncture has a role in relieving the pain of individual joints but should not replace orthodox treatment which can slow down the progression of the disease.

Likelihood of being helped by acupuncture ●●●

Tennis elbow (the medical name for this is lateral epicondylitis) is a painful condition caused by damage to the muscles and tendons of the outside of the elbow and forearm. Though it can be caused by playing tennis, it usually isn't and there is often no obvious cause. Repetitive use of the elbow may trigger a tennis elbow.

My clinical experience suggests that the majority of people suffering from tennis elbow can be helped by acupuncture – sometimes dramatically. This is supported by the scientific research which confirms that acupuncture effectively relieves the pain of tennis elbow, certainly in the short-term, and may be more effective than other treatments such as ultrasound therapy.[12]

There is a related condition colloquially known as 'golfer's elbow' which is less common and affects the other – inner – side of the elbow joint. A patient who came to see me called Gordon actually did get his golfer's elbow from playing golf, though, as with tennis elbow, most sufferers do not play golf. Gordon, a 58 year old chief executive, had recently started playing golf again after a reduction in his work commitments. This had caused him to feel a pain around the inside of his right elbow that was made worse with certain swings such as hitting the ground with his club. Taking anti-inflammatory painkillers helped relieve the pain but he was hoping for a more permanent cure. He had a classic golfer's elbow with tenderness around the inside of the elbow joint (medical epicondylitis). I gave him just three acupuncture treatments, focusing on a combination of trigger points around the affected area, 'periosteal pecking' (a rather uncomfortable – but sometimes very effective – technique of tapping the surface of the bone with the acupuncture needle) and using a couple of nearby traditional acupuncture points. By the third treatment, Gordon felt 'really good indeed.' ' I'm really pleased', he told me. He said that his pain was 95 per cent gone, and that was despite having played two rounds of golf the previous weekend. We agreed that we would stop there for now and that he would return for top-up treatments if his pain recurred. Not everyone responds as well as Gordon did, but his story does demonstrate how well acupuncture can help relieve a condition that is, traditionally, very difficult to treat.

I find that between 6 and 10 treatments, given once or twice weekly, are usually required to provide maximum benefit.

Likelihood of being helped by acupuncture ●●●

RSI is the name given to a group of injuries affecting the muscles, tendons and nerves of, mainly, the hands, arms and neck. It is also known as 'work related upper limb disorder'. Tennis and golfer's elbow are examples of RSI though there are many different types. RSI can be a particularly stubborn problem that is difficult to treat. Sometimes the only solution is for complete rest of the affected area, which can be very frustrating for those who are then unable to work.

My experience tells me that acupuncture can have a lot to offer especially if treatment is not delayed too long. Once pain is felt continuously the problem becomes far more difficult to treat and the road to recovery can be long.

This is another condition, like most musculoskeletal problems, that I find best suited to treatment with a western style of acupuncture concentrating on tight knots of muscle in the affected area known as Trigger Points.

Likelihood of being helped by acupuncture ●● to ●●●● depending on severity and length of time of condition

Fibromyalgia is a long-term condition causing widespread musculoskeletal pain ('pain all over'), fatigue, poor sleep, bowel symptoms, headaches and other symptoms. The cause is unknown and treatments are geared towards relieving symptoms and are often unsatisfactory. Though research suggests that acupuncture offers little apart from some pain relief (which in itself is not to be scoffed at), some patients clearly respond to acupuncture and so, in the absence of other good treatments, it is worth a trial.[13]

Patients with fibromyalgia are more likely to suffer from a temporary aggravation of pain following treatment than most other patients receiving acupuncture. For this reason many acupuncturists are cautious about needling the tender points, either avoiding needling them directly and inserting needles nearby instead or needling for a very brief time, maybe no more than 30 seconds. For those who tolerate treatment, electro-acupuncture may be the most effective form of treatment.

Likelihood of being helped by acupuncture ●●

There is little evidence to support the use of acupuncture for *frozen shoulder* (adhesive capsulitis). My experience – both as an acupuncturist and a patient – is that acupuncture has little to offer. Having said that, it is such a painful condition, that anything that might help, including acupuncture, is worth a try.[14]

Likelihood of being helped by acupuncture ○

Acupuncture may be able to hasten the healing of muscle strains, sprains and sports injuries.

Likelihood of being helped by acupuncture ●●●

1   Haake M et al. German Acupuncture Trials (GERAC) for Chronic Low Back Pain. Archives of Internal Medicine 2007; 167(17): 1892-1898.

2   Furlan AD et al. Acupuncture and dry-needling for low back pain, Cochrane Database of Systematic Reviews 2005, Issue 1. Art. No.: CD001351. DOI: 10.1002/14651858.CD001351.pub2.

3   Ernst E, White A. Acupuncture for back pain: A meta-analysis of randomized controlled trials. Archives of Internal Medicine 1998; 158: 2235-2241.

4   Low Back Pain: early management of persistent non-specific low back pain. NICE clinical guideline 88; May 2009.

5   Irnich D et al. Randomised trial of acupuncture compared with massage and 'sham' laser acupuncture for treatment of chronic neck pain. BMJ 2001; 322: 1-6

6   Itoh K et al. Randomised trial of trigger point acupuncture compared with other acupuncture for treatment of chronic neck pain. Complementary Therapies in Medicine 2007; 15:172-9.

7   David J et al. Chronic neck pain: a comparison of acupuncture treatment and physiotherapy. British Journal of Rheumatology 1998; 37: 1118-1122.

8   Kwon YD, Pittler MH, Ernst E. Acupuncture for peripheral joint osteoarthritis. A systematic review and meta-analysis. Rheumatology 2006; 45: 1331-1337.

9   White A, Foster NE, Cummings M, Barlas P. Acupuncture treatment for chronic knee pain: a systematic review. Rheumatology 2007; 46: 384-90.

10   Choi TY et al. Moxibustion for rheumatic conditions: a systematic review and meta-analysis. Clin Rheumatol. 2011; 30(7): 937-45.

11   Christensen BV, Iuhl IU, Vilbek H, Bülow H-H, Dreijer NC, Rasmussen HF. Acupuncture treatment of severe knee osteoarthrosis. A long-term study. Acta Anaesthesiologica Scandinavica 1992; 36: 519-525.

12   Trinh KV et al. Acupuncture for the alleviation of lateral epicondyle pain: a systematic review. Rheumatology 2004; 43: 1085-90.

13   Langhorst J et al. Efficacy of acupuncture in fibromyalgia syndrome a systematic review with a meta-analysis of controlled clinical trials. Rheumatology 2010; 49: 778-88.

14   Green S et al. Acupuncture for shoulder pain. Cochrane Database Syst Rev 2005; 18: CD005319.

7

Headaches & Migraines

All of us have suffered a bad headache on at least one occasion. In most cases a couple of paracetamol tablets, a Nurofen or a good night's sleep sorts things out. However for some people headaches can be a regular and disabling occurrence. Before seeking any treatment, lifestyle issues should first be examined: drinking too much coffee or not enough liquids are common causes of headaches as are stress, depression and skipping meals.

There are many causes of headaches; some of these respond well to acupuncture.

The most common type of headache is so-called *'tension' headache*, usually resulting in a pressing or tightening pain over both sides of the head.

I find that acupuncture is most likely to be effective when these headaches are the result of muscular tension. When this is the case, then treating the tense areas of muscle, especially over the neck and top of the shoulders, can help relieve the pain.

Because there are so many different causes of headache, researching the effects of treatment is difficult; nevertheless, the best research does suggest that 'acupuncture could be a valuable option for patients suffering from frequent tension-like headaches'.[1] Clinical experience tells us that acupuncture can be a very useful treatment in many, but not all, patients. Acupuncture is usually more helpful in prevention rather than relieving a headache currently being experienced.

Likelihood of being helped by acupuncture ●●●

I find acupuncture extremely effective for *migraine*, with most sufferers obtaining significant relief with a large reduction in the frequency of attacks.

My clinical experience is supported by the research evidence which shows that acupuncture is more effective than conventional drug treatment for migraine and gives less side-effects (acupuncture actually has extremely few side-effects).[2]

Linda, a 40 year old PA, had suffered from migraines and headaches for many years. She had been to see a neurologist who arranged an MRI scan which, much to her relief, was normal. Her specialist referred Linda to me for a course of acupuncture treatment. When I saw her, she was experiencing daily headaches in addition to migraines once or twice a month. She also had pain over the top of her shoulders. When I examined Linda I found her to be very tender in the muscles of her neck and over her shoulders. I treated Linda's numerous 'trigger points' (painful knots of muscle) in her neck and shoulder area. This is a western style of acupuncture treatment that does not utilize traditional Chinese medical theory. After four treatments, Linda was completely free of headaches. She agreed to return for 'top-up' treatments if her headaches returned.

Treatment usually involves 6-8 weekly treatments after which the gap between treatments can usually be extended. Sometimes long-term, but infrequent, treatment may be necessary to keep the migraines away.

Likelihood of being helped by acupuncture ●●●●.

Notes to chapter 7

1 Melchart D et al. Acupuncture for idiopathic headache. Cochrane Database of Systematic Reviews 2001, Issue 1. Art.No: CD0011218. DOI: 10.1002/14651858.CD001218.

2 Linde K, Allais G, Brinkhaus B, Manheimer E, Vickers A, White AR. Acupuncture for tension-type headache. Cochrane Database of Systematic Reviews 2009, Issue 1. Art. No.: CD007587. DOI: 10.1002/14651858.CD07587

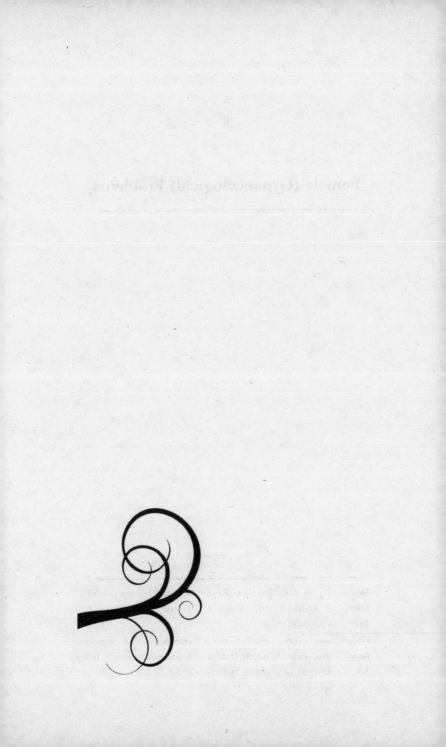

8

Female (Gynaecological) Problems

I have been treating women suffering from *period pain* (dysmenorrhoea) with acupuncture for many years and it has often appeared to help. So I was pleased to see a recent large research paper looking at all the trials done on the use of acupuncture in period pain and finding that it was not only effective at relieving period pain but appeared to be more effective than the commonly used anti-inflammatory painkillers most often prescribed by GPs.[1]

There is even some scientific logic as to why acupuncture might work in this condition: needles are placed in the lower abdomen and stimulate the spinal cord in the same area that also connects to the womb, and can thus exert an effect on the womb in ways we do not fully understand.

I usually recommend weekly treatments for the first couple of months after which the treatment interval can be extended depending on the response to treatment. Needles are usually inserted in the lower abdomen, legs and feet.

Likelihood of being helped by acupuncture ●●●●

Some women sail through the *menopause* (change of life) without blinking an eye. But most women experience some unpleasant symptoms and, for some, the experience can be both distressing and disabling. Hot flushes and night sweats are the most common problems at this time of life but sleep disturbance, irritability, inability to concentrate, vaginal dryness and urinary problems can all occur. During the 1980s and 1990s, oestrogen – or hormone – replacement therapy (HRT) was widely promoted and prescribed as a panacea for the menopause. Women, and doctors, were advised that this not only relieved women of their disturbing symptoms but was also good for them in numerous other ways including preventing heart disease, osteoporosis (thinning of the bones) and dementia. This was all accompanied by aggressive marketing campaigns by the pharmaceutical companies who could see a windfall coming their way. We are now older and wiser. We now know that the use of HRT, especially for long periods, increases the risk of breast cancer, cancer of the ovaries, heart disease and blood clots (thromboses). Women now often look to complementary therapies as an alternative to HRT.

Research shows that acupuncture does have an effect on menopausal hot flushes, giving women significant relief. However, how it does this is uncertain. Proponents of traditional Chinese medicine argue that these beneficial effects arise from rebalancing the energy as it flows through the body's meridians. However, modern scientific research suggests that it may influence the temperature regulating centre in the brain by its effect on neuro-chemicals in the brain.[2]

My clinical impression is that some women are greatly helped by acupuncture treatment based on traditional Chinese principles. Kate is a good example. I first met Kate when she was 50 years old and had been going through the change for 4 months. She was tired and moody, fluctuating between feeling tearful and irritable. To add insult to injury she had also put on weight. She suffered from the typical menopausal symptoms: she was woken up three times a night with night sweats and had half a dozen episodes of hot flushes daily. She loved using saunas but this had become impossible as it was sure to bring her out in a horrendous hot flush.

Kate was a fit, active lady and had already tried yoga, exercise and meditation along with the herbal remedies Agnus Castus and Starflower. By the time she came to see me she was desperate for help.

We agreed on a course of six weekly treatments in the first instance. I treated Kate using traditional Chinese principles, inserting needles into points in her legs, arms and head. After six treatments she was feeling much improved, but still had some symptoms, and so we decided to continue treatment in order to maintain the improvement. After nine treatments Kate told me she was 95 per cent better, no longer waking at all at night and only getting mild flushes during the day. We agreed to decrease the frequency of the treatments to one every 2-3 weeks.

Kate remained well apart from one episode of recurrence of symptoms during a five week period without treatment. And she was able to visit the sauna again regularly.

Treatment for menopausal symptoms is usually given for several months, initially weekly and later less frequently.

Likelihood of being helped by acupuncture ●●●

Polycystic Ovarian Syndrome (PCOS) is the most common female hormone disorder. It can cause irregular periods, infertility and excessive hair growth. PCOS increases the risk of developing diabetes and hypertension (high blood pressure).

Mary, aged 30, had suffered from PCOS for ten years and had been trying to conceive – unsuccessfully – for the last three years. Her periods were pretty irregular, as is usual with PCOS, usually occurring every 4-8 weeks. As well as her problems conceiving, Mary also suffered from excessive hair growth, weight gain and spots on her skin. I treated her weekly for six weeks using traditional acupuncture points on her feet, legs, abdomen and arms. The seventh time I saw her she was beaming as she told me she was pregnant. We will, of course, never know for certain whether acupuncture helped her conceive or not, though Mary certainly felt it contributed.

Though there is little research on the use of acupuncture in PCOS, there is good reason to believe that acupuncture could be a useful support to help induce ovulation, and may also relieve other symptoms without causing the common side-effects of orthodox medication.[3] There is now research that suggests that a course of electro-acupuncture may produce long-lasting beneficial effects in women with PCOS who are unable to ovulate (produce eggs). This may be a result of acupuncture stimulating the hypothalamus and pituitary gland in the base of the brain. These areas of the brain are responsible for the release of hormones that influence fertility and menstruation.

Likelihood of being helped by acupuncture ●●

There has been a lot of publicity over recent years surrounding the use of acupuncture to help women conceive.

There have been numerous reports of women who have managed to conceive following acupuncture treatment. There is some scientific research that supports the plausibility of this: for example, electro-acupuncture to the lower abdomen increases the blood flow to the womb (uterus) and acupuncture has been shown to trigger the release in the brain of the hormones governing *fertility*, both of which could aid conception.

Most of the scientific research has concentrated on the use of acupuncture as an aid to conception using in vitro fertilisation (IVF).

A systematic review and meta-analysis (considered the highest level of evidence based medicine) published in the British Medical Journal in 2008 concluded 'acupuncture given with embryo transfer improved rates of pregnancy and live birth among women undergoing in vitro fertilisation'.[4] Other research has found that ear acupuncture is as effective as hormonal treatment in helping women conceive.[5] Acupuncture may work by increasing the blood flow to the womb and ovaries and by its effect on female hormones.[6]

Paula, a 37 year old events manager, had been trying to conceive for over a year. She was in the process of having investigations at the fertility clinic, all of which had been normal. After two treatments of traditional Chinese acupuncture she conceived. I would like to think that the acupuncture had a part to play in baby Zak's entry into the world nine months later.

Likelihood of being helped by acupuncture ●●● (●●●● if associated with IVF)

Endometriosis is a strange condition in which endometrial tissue (material from the womb) grows in parts of the body other than the womb, most commonly on the ovaries, tubes or other organs in the pelvis. The condition most often causes pain, especially at the time of menstruation, but can also cause painful intercourse and infertility. The treatment usually involves surgical excision of the unwanted tissue or treatment of the symptoms with medication.

There is limited evidence to think acupuncture may help some women with endometriosis, with pain being the symptom that is probably most likely to be helped.[7] A course of 6-8 treatments should be sufficient to know whether acupuncture is likely to help or not.

Likelihood of being helped by acupuncture ●●

Most women experience *premenstrual symptoms* at some stage in their lives and for 1 in 10 women the symptoms are bad enough to disrupt their daily lives. PMS causes symptoms that are both physical (breast tenderness, abdominal bloating, headaches, swollen ankles) and psychological (irritability, mood swings, loss of temper, spontaneous crying, poor concentration).

Most women notice a gradual worsening of symptoms in the week leading up to their period. Symptoms usually fade rapidly once menstruation starts, though they can persist throughout menstruation in some women. This specific relationship in time to the menstrual cycle distinguishes PMS from other conditions that can cause similar symptoms such as depression, stress or thyroid disorders. Conventional treatments for PMS include hormonal treatments such as progestogens and the contraceptive pill, vitamin B6 and symptomatic treatments such as diuretics (water tablets) and antidepressants.

Though one study has found acupuncture to be better than Premarin tablets (a hormonal treatment) at relieving PMS symptoms, there is insufficient research to be sure what role acupuncture has to play in the widespread treatment of PMS. My clinical impression is that acupuncture helps some, but by no means all, women. Treatment – once or twice a week – over two months is sufficient to judge whether acupuncture is helping, though it is sometimes necessary to continue treatment for many months, though usually at longer intervals, such as monthly.[8,9]

Likelihood of being helped by acupuncture ●●

1 Cho S-H, Hwang E-W. Acupuncture for primary dysmenorrhoea: a systematic review. British Journal of Obstetrics and Gynaecology 2010; 117: 509-521

2 Borud E, White A. A review of acupuncture for menopausal problems. Maturitas 2010; 66: 131-4.

3 Stener-Victorin E, Jedel E, Mannerås L. Acupuncture in polycystic Ovarian Syndrome: Current Experimental and Clinical Evidence. Journal of Neuroendocrinology 2008; 20: 290-8.

4 Manheimer E. Zhang G. Udoff L. Haramati A. Langenberg P. Berman BM. Bouter LM. Effects of acupuncture on rates of pregnancy and live birth among women undergoing in vitro fertilisation: systematic review and meta-analysis. BMJ 2008; 336(7643):545-9.

5 Gergard J, Postneek F. Auricular acupuncture in the treatment of female infertility. Gynaecological Endocrinology 1992; 6(3): 171-81.

6 Stener-Victorin E, Humaidan P. Use of acupuncture in female infertility and a summary of recent acupuncture studies related to embryo transfer. Acupuncture in Medicine 2006; 24(4): 157-163.

7 Wayne PM et al. Japanese-style acupuncture for endometriosis-related pelvic pain in adolescents and young women: results of a randomized sham-controlled trial. J Pediatr Adolesc Gynecol 2008; 21(5): 247-57.

8 Jin H et al. Clinical observation on acupuncture at the five-zangshu for treatment of perimenopausal syndrome. [Chinese]. Zhongguo Zhenjiu 2007; 27:572-4.

9 Cho SH, Kim J. Efficacy of acupuncture in management of premenstrual syndrome: A systematic review. Complementary Therapies in Medicine 2010; 18: 104-11

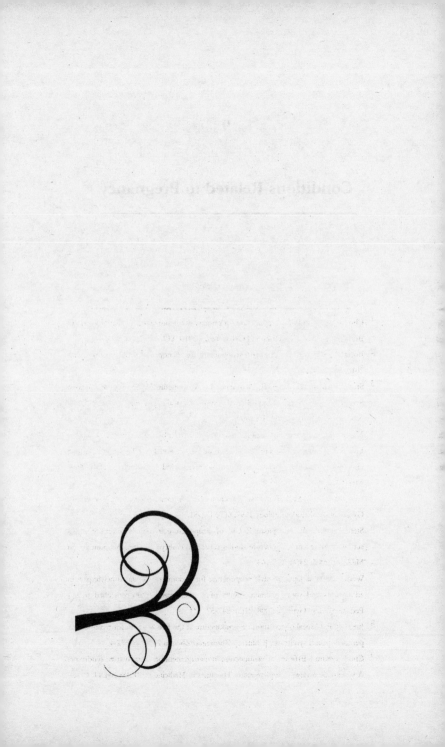

9

Conditions Related to Pregnancy

Surprisingly, there is more scientific evidence supporting the use of acupuncture to treat nausea and vomiting than for any other condition. The nausea and vomiting of pregnancy ('hyperemesis gravidum' or *morning sickness*) is no exception. Acupuncture using traditional Chinese principles relieves the 'morning sickness' of early pregnancy.[1] The treatment usually centres around one point on the forearm a little above the wrist called Neiguan (meaning Inner Pass) and also known as point PC6. There is no rational Western explanation why needling this particular point should relieve nausea and vomiting but lots of research and clinical experience confirm its effectiveness. Though point PC6 will almost certainly be used, other points may be needled as well. Treatment is usually given several times a week and usually works within a week.

Likelihood of being helped by acupuncture ●●●●●

One of the more remarkable effects of acupuncture is its ability to turn around a baby that is positioned bottom first inside the womb, or in a *'breech presentation'*.

Even more remarkable is that the most effective treatment involves needling or, even more improbably, holding a stick of burning moxa (a Chinese herb – *See chapter 2*) over an acu-point on the tip of the little toe known as Bladder 67 or 'Zhi Yin' meaning 'reaching yin'.

Nevertheless, numerous studies have confirmed that this treatment works.[2]

The best time to use acupuncture to attempt to turn a breech presentation is probably between the 32nd and 35th weeks of pregnancy. Frequent treatments are required, ideally daily, but when the herbal moxa sticks are used, the expectant mother can use these to treat herself.

Likelihood of being helped by acupuncture ●●●●

Heartburn, upper abdominal pain, belching and bloating are all common but unwanted symptoms of pregnancy. Heartburn, felt as a burning pain in the middle of the chest or in the pit of the stomach, is the most common of these.

Acupuncture seems to be an effective treatment for heartburn in pregnant women.[3]

Treatment is usually given weekly until the symptoms have been relieved; this usually takes between 4 and 6 treatments. The most commonly used points are in the upper abdomen and in the legs.

Likelihood of being helped by acupuncture ●●●●

Low back pain is a common problem in pregnant women. Acupuncture is well recognised as an effective treatment for low back pain in the general population. So it is not surprising that acupuncture has also been found to help relieve the *low back pain* and *pelvic pain* suffered by pregnant women.[4,5]

Likelihood of being helped by acupuncture ●●●●

Acupuncture can also help relieve the pain of child-birth, though it may not always be easy or practicable to have an acupuncturist available and have needles inserted during *labour*. Acupuncture may also help to induce labour: it may shorten the duration of labour by between 12 and 24 hours.

Likelihood of being helped by acupuncture ●●.

Notes to chapter 9

1   Smith C, Crowther C, Beilby J. Acupuncture to treat nausea and vomiting in early pregnancy: a randomized controlled trial. Birth 2002; 29: 1-9.

2   van den Berg I, Bosch JL, Jacobs B, Bouman I, Duvekot JJ, Hunink MGM. Effectiveness of acupuncture-type interventions versus expectant management to correct breech presentation: A systematic review. Complementary Therapies in Medicine 2008; 16: 92-100.

3   da Silva JBG, Nakamura MU, Cordeiro JA, Kulay L, Saidah R. Acupuncture for dyspepsia in pregnancy: a prospective, randomised controlled study. Acupuncture in Medicine 2009; 27: 50-53.

4   Elden H, Ladfors L, Olsen MF, Ostgaard H-C, Hagberg H. Effects of acupuncture and stabilising exercises as adjunct to standard treatment in pregnant women with pelvic girdle pain: randomised single blind controlled trial. BMJ, doi.10.1136/bmj.38397.507014.E0.

5   Wand S-M, DeZine P, Lin EC, Lin H, Yue JJ, Berman MR, Braveman F, Kain ZN. Auricular acupuncture as a treatment for pregnant women who have low back and posterior pelvic pain: a pilot study. American Journal of Obstetrics & Gynaecology 2009; 271: e1-9

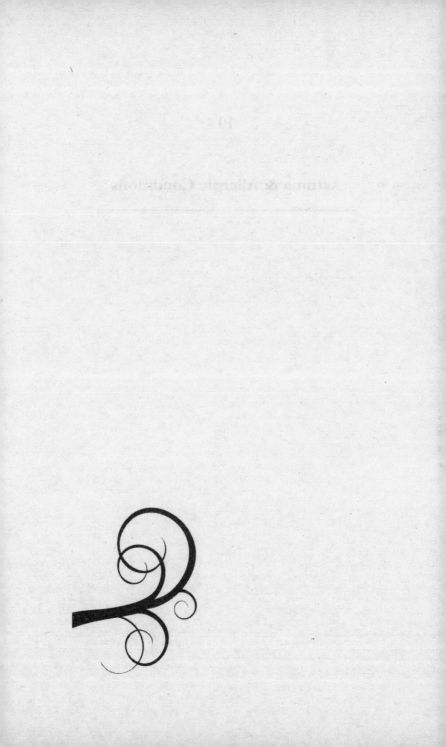

10

Asthma & Allergic Conditions

Asthma is a common condition that affects the airways – the tubes that carry air from the nose and mouth into the lungs. It causes these tubes to become narrow and inflamed resulting in the typical symptoms of shortness of breath, wheezing and cough. Though many sufferers have quite mild asthma, possibly triggered only by exercise, an infection or by coming into contact with something they are allergic to, three people still die every day from asthma in the UK. Most treatment involves using inhalers or 'puffers', either regularly as a preventive or used occasionally when symptoms occur.

Though the evidence on the use of acupuncture in asthma is somewhat confusing and contradictory, many acupuncturists, especially those using traditional Chinese acupuncture, report dramatic successes.

Asthma is – at least in part – an immune-related disorder and it is possible that acupuncture can affect the immune system in some individuals to prevent attacks.

Clinical experience suggests that acupuncture can help some people with asthma but that others are not helped. This would not be surprising because asthma is not a uniform disease but is really a description of symptoms which have a wide variety of different causes.[1] As asthma can be life-threatening, medication should not be stopped during acupuncture treatment without medical approval.

The bottom line is that acupuncture may help some people with asthma but regular treatments may be needed for many months.

Likelihood of being helped by acupuncture ●●

Hay fever is caused by an allergy to the pollen from grasses, trees, plants and – perhaps not surprisingly – hay. It affects people during the pollen season in the spring and summer and causes a runny or blocked nose, itchy and watery eyes and a sore itchy throat. Standard treatments involving eye drops, nasal sprays and anti-histamine tablets are often very effective. However they do not relieve the symptoms in everyone and some people look to alternative treatments for additional relief.

Clinical experience tells us that people suffering from hay fever can be helped by acupuncture, sometimes dramatically. This impression is supported by some scientific research.[2,3] Twice-weekly treatments are sometimes needed during the hay fever season when symptoms are at their worst. Between 3 and 6 weekly treatments before the hay fever season starts may prevent attacks altogether. Needles are usually inserted in the face, legs and arms.

Likelihood of being helped by acupuncture ●●●

Clinical experience suggests that acupuncture may be particularly useful in allergic conditions of the skin such as *urticaria*. This is supported by studies demonstrating an anti-histamine effect of acupuncture.[4,5] It is possible that acupuncture works here in a similar way to taking an anti-histamine tablet.

Likelihood of being helped by acupuncture ●●

Notes to chapter 10

---

1 White A, Cummings M, Filshie J, Eds. An Introduction to Western Medical Acupuncture. Churchill Livingstone 2008.

2 Ng DK et al. A double-blind randomized placebo-controlled trial of acupuncture for the treatment of childhood persistent allergic rhinitis. Pediatrics 2004; 114: 1242-7.

3 Xue CCL et al. Acupuncture for persistent allergic rhinitis: a randomised, sham-controlled trial. Medical Journal of Australia 2007; 187: 337-41.

4 Belgrade MJ, Solomon LM, Lichter EA. Effect of acupuncture on experimentally induced itch. Acta Dermatologica Venereologica 1084; 64: 129-33.

5 Lundeberg T, Bondesson L, Thomas M. Effect of acupuncture on experimentally induced itch. British Journal of Dermatology 1987; 117: 771-7.

11

Addictions

Acupuncture has been a popular treatment for addictions for many years and is used all over the world for this purpose. The reason it can help addictions may be because it stimulates areas of the brain – and certain neuro-chemicals – that reduce pain, stress and anxiety and help promote relaxation.

The type of acupuncture usually used is ear acupuncture (also called auriculotherapy – See chapter 2), sometimes with electric stimulation during the treatment.

In addition, tiny needles are sometimes left in the ear between treatments as there is some evidence that this may be the most effective form of acupuncture for treating substance misuse and may be more effective than other interventions such as hyp-notherapy. Because of the small but serious risk of infection from these 'indwelling' needles, I prefer to use small metal balls which are held in place over the acu-points with sticky plaster.

Clinical trials have demonstrated a positive effect of acupuncture on people who want to *stop smoking*.[1,2,3]

A recent rigorous systematic review and meta-analysis that combines all high quality trials (the 'highest' form of evidence based medicine) has confirmed the benefit of acupuncture in helping those trying to give up tobacco. Acupuncture was found to have a significant benefit in helping people stop smoking immediately after a course of treatment and at both three and six months following treatment. Acupuncture showed maximum benefit three months after the completion of a course of treatment, when those treated with acupuncture were two and a half times more likely to have stopped smoking than those who received other treatments.[4]

My own view based on clinical experience is that acupuncture can indeed be a useful support to those wanting to stop smoking provided that the willpower is there. In other words, it will not do the job for you – you still have to do much of the hard work but acupuncture can make the effort that bit easier.

Treatment usually involves having needles inserted into the ear and sometimes other areas as well.

Likelihood of being helped by acupuncture ●●●

Acupuncture can help suppress the effects of withdrawal from *opiates* such as heroin, morphine and codeine.[5] It may also help with withdrawal from other drugs such as *cocaine* and *alcohol*. The science is not encouraging but many trials miss the point of what acupuncture has to offer in alcohol and drug rehabilitation. The most helpful aspect of acupuncture may be simply to calm addicts so that they can continue with abstinence and any withdrawal programmes more comfortably. Clinical use suggests that addicts become more relaxed with a more positive outlook and are able to abstain with less difficulty with the support of acupuncture.

One commonly used protocol involves inserting five tiny needles in each ear and leaving them in for up to an hour during each treatment session. People are often treated in groups and acupuncture should always be combined with other supportive treatments including counseling and education.

Likelihood of being helped by acupuncture ●●● (when given as part of a comprehensive therapeutic package)

Research suggests acupuncture is a safe and effective treatment for *obesity*. Various forms of acupuncture may help, including ear and electro-acupuncture.[6] The stimulation of ear acupuncture points has been shown to suppress appetite. In one trial over three quarters of those who received stimulation of acupuncture points lost over 2Kg in weight over the 12-week treatment period.[7] Treatment at least once weekly, and preferably more frequently, for at least two months, is likely to be necessary to result in significant weight loss. Inevitably successful weight loss is far more likely to be achieved if acupuncture is combined with dietary and lifestyle changes.

Likelihood of being helped by acupuncture ●●●

Notes to chapter 11

1 He D. Medbo JI. Hostmark AT. Effect of acupuncture on smoking cessation or reduction: an 8-month and 5-year follow-up study. Preventive Medicine 2001; 33(5):364-72.

2 Dong H, Berg JE, Høstmark AT. Effects of acupuncture on smoking cessation or reduction for motivated smokers. Preventive Medicine 1997; 26: 208-214.

3 Waite N, Clough JB. A single-blind, placebo-controlled trial of a simple acupuncture treatment in the cessation of smoking. British Journal of General Practice 1998; 48: 1487-1490.

4 Cheng HM, Chung YC, Chen HH, Chang YH, Yeh ML. Systematic Review and Meta-Analysis of the effects of Acupoint Stimulation on Smoking Cessation. American Journal of Clinical Medicine 2012; 40(3): 429-442.

5 Clement-Jones V, McLoughlin L, Besser GM, Rees LH, Wen HL. Acupuncture in heroin addicts; changes in Met-enkephalin and beta-endorphin in blood and cerebrospinal fluid. Lancet 1979; 2(8139): 380-3.

6 Cho SH et al. Acupuncture for obesity: a systematic review and meta-analysis. International Journal of Obesity (Lond). 2009 Feb;33(2):183-96.

7 Richards D, Marley J. Stimulation of auricular acupuncture points in weight loss. Australian Family Physician 1998; 27 Suppl 2: S73-7.

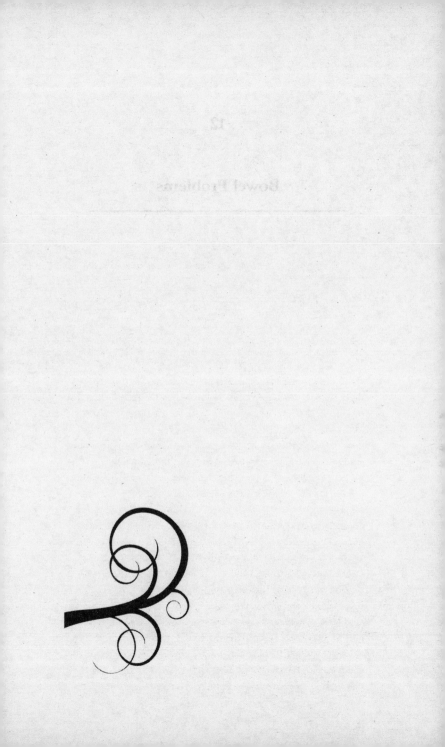

12

Bowel Problems

Irritable Bowel Syndrome (IBS) is a distressing condition that, at its worst, can ruin the sufferer's quality of life. It manifests itself differently in patient to patient, but usually results in some or all of the following: recurrent abdominal pain, bloating, constipation and diarrhoea. There is no satisfactory medical treatment; the best modern drugs can do no more than alleviate some of the symptoms.

Rachel, a 28 year old business manager at a large City bank, had suffered from IBS for many years. She was plagued with symptoms of diarrhoea, low abdominal cramping and bloating. She had to open her bowels an average of five times a day. This was making her life very difficult and was causing her considerable anxiety which was, in turn, aggravating her symptoms. She was caught in a vicious spiral. 'It's ruining my life right now', were her very words when I first met her. After six acupuncture treatments, given at weekly intervals, Rachel's symptoms were much improved; she no longer had any cramping or bloating, and opened her bowels up to a maximum of three times a day, sometimes going a whole day without having to go to the toilet – a new, and welcome, experience for her. She remains well with occasional top-up treatments.

From the scientific viewpoint, a few trials have found that sufferers have been helped with acupuncture treatment, though it may be that the placebo effect plays a significant part in this improvement.[1,2]

My own clinical impression is that around half of those I have treated are very much helped by acupuncture.

Likelihood of being helped by acupuncture ●●●

Inflammatory bowel disease, of which the two most common are ulcerative colitis (UC) and Crohn's disease (CD), can cause abdominal cramps and pain, diarrhoea (often severe and mixed with blood) and sometimes fever and weight loss. Drugs are usually taken to suppress the symptoms and occasionally surgery is required to remove severely affected parts of the bowel.

Though Chinese researchers have concluded that acupuncture is a safe and effective (and even better than western medicine) treatment for ulcerative colitis, this is not generally accepted in the West.[3] However, there is limited research which suggests that acupuncture can help sufferers of both UC and CD by reducing the disease activity and increasing the quality of life and well being of sufferers.[4]

I have been seeing Vladimir for many years. The 59 year old artist has suffered from UC for as long as I, and probably he, can remember. Like most sufferers he goes for periods with very little in the way of symptoms, but then gets flare ups, sometimes brought on by a stressful life event. He is under the hospital specialist and takes medication when advised to. Vladimir asked me some 20 years ago, at a time when his symptoms were bad, whether acupuncture might help him as he preferred not to take medication if he didn't have to. I told him that it might help, but that I couldn't make any promises; if he wished we could try and see. Vladimir wanted to give it a go and so I gave him an initial six week course of treatment. To his delight his symptoms improved a fair bit during treatment. Ever since then he has returned every now and then, once a year on average, to have a brief course of 2 or 3 treatments when he has a flare up. He is quite sure that it helps, so sure in fact that he gave me one of his paintings as a thank you.

Likelihood of being helped by acupuncture ●●

Notes to chapter 12

1 Chan J. The role of acupuncture in the treatment of irritable bowel syndrome: a pilot study. Hepato-Gastroenterology 1997; 44:1328-1330.

2 SchneiderA et al. Acupuncture treatment in irritable bowel syndrome. 2006; 55: 649-654.

3 Mu JP et al. Meta-analysis on acupuncture and moxibustion for treatment of ulcerative colitis. [Chinese]. Zhongguo Zhenjiu 2007; 27: 687-90.

4 Schneider A, Streitberger K, Joos S. Acupuncture treatment in gastrointestinal diseases: A systematic review. World Journal of Gastroenterology 2007; 13(25): 3417-3424.

13

Psychological problems

In Traditional Chinese Medicine (TCM), the heart (that is the 'Chinese' heart which is not the same as what we think of as the heart in western medicine) is believed to be the main organ that 'governs' our mental state. Any TCM acupuncture treatment of psychological or emotional symptoms is likely to include points along the heart meridian running down the arm. A Western explanation for any positive effect acupuncture may have on our emotional well-being is more likely to focus on acupuncture's effect on our neurotransmitters, the chemicals that take messages from one brain cell to the next.

Patients often tell me that they feel relaxed after an acupuncture treatment. So one might think that acupuncture could be used helpfully to relax or to relieve anxiety and stress.

In clinical practice I do find that acupuncture can help reduce *anxiety* and even help patients *sleep better*. I have to admit that not everyone is helped with acupuncture in this regard, but some certainly are.

One trial suggests that acupuncture may help adults suffering from chronic *stress*, though the authors acknowledged that stress is extremely difficult to measure.[1]

There has unfortunately been very little research into the effects of acupuncture on anxiety and sleep. However, one small study found a marked improvement in the quality and length of sleep, accompanied by a reduction in stress, in adults who received acupuncture twice weekly for five weeks.[2] Interestingly, a scientific basis for acupuncture's positive effect was found in this study: those treated with acupuncture were found to have increased levels of melatonin at night. Melatonin is a naturally occurring compound that helps induce sleep and regulate the sleep-wake cycle; body levels of melatonin are naturally higher during the night.

A thorough review of all trials on acupuncture and insomnia concluded that acupuncture may help improve sleep but criticised the quality of the trials.[3]

Likelihood of being helped by acupuncture ●●

Depression is extremely common with two thirds of adults experiencing depression severe enough to interfere with their normal activities at some stage in their lives. In Britain, depression is estimated to cost £7.5 billion a year in medication, benefits and lost working days.

A number of studies from China have concluded that acupuncture is a safe and effective treatment for depression working at least as well as Western antidepressant medication but with less side-effects.[4] However, these studies have been criticised and it has been suggested that the apparent positive benefit from acupuncture is largely a placebo affect (though antidepressant drugs are also known to have a large placebo effect).[5]

My clinical impression is that acupuncture can be a helpful supportive treatment for people suffering from mild to moderate depression but that it should be used alongside other treatments particularly talking treatments such as counseling, CBT or psychotherapy.

No treatment will have a substantial influence on depression if there are lifestyle issues that are causing the problem in the first place that are not being addressed. However, the real effectiveness of anti-depressant medication has been questioned and since it can cause significant side-effects

including difficulty stopping the tablets, it seems
reasonable for sufferers to look elsewhere for help.

Likelihood of being helped by acupuncture ●●

Notes to chapter 13

---

1   Huang W et al. An investigation into the effectiveness of traditional Chinese acupuncture (TCA) for chronic stress in adults: a randomised controlled pilot study. Complement Ther Clin Pract 2011; 17: 16-21.

2   Spence DW, Kayumov L, Chen A et al. Acupuncture increases nocturnal melatonin secretion and reduces insomnia and anxiety: a preliminary report. Journal of Neuropsychiatry and Clinical Neurosciences 2004; 16: 19-28

3   Cheuk DK et al. Acupuncture for insomnia. Cochrane Database Syst Rev 2007; 18: CD005472.

4   Zhang Z.-J et al. The effectiveness and safety of acupuncture therapy in depressive disorders: Systematic review and meta-analysis. Journal of Affective Disorders. 2010;124 (1-2) (pp 9-21).

5   Ernst E, Lee MS, Choi TY Acupuncture for Depression? A Systematic Review of Systematic Reviews. Eval Health Prof. 2010 Dec 7. doi: 10.1177/0163278710386109.

14

Cancer

There are dozens of different types of cancer which vary widely in how easy – or difficult – they are to treat and how likely they are to be cured. There is no evidence that acupuncture can cure cancer and it should not be used for that aim, particularly if this prevents the cancer patient from seeking medical help that is potentially curative or, at least more appropriate.

However, cancer does cause a myriad of symptoms, such as fatigue and pain, some of which can be helped by acupuncture.

Pain

This is one of the most common symptoms of cancer and one which some people fear the most. Though there are effective pain relieving drugs, all have side-effects. Nearly everyone with advanced cancer suffers some pain and many do not get sufficient pain relief. One of acupuncture's primary uses is for pain relief and there is limited evidence to suggest that acupuncture may provide long-term pain relief in cancer sufferers.[1]

Likelihood of being helped by acupuncture ●●●

Fatigue

Fatigue is the most common symptom reported by cancer survivors and can be debilitating. Acupuncture may help reduce the fatigue in some, though the evidence for this is not strong, possibly because there have only been a few small trials done.[2]

Likelihood of being helped by acupuncture ●●

Dry mouth (xerostomia)

Dry mouth is a common side-effect of having radiotherapy for a cancer of the head or neck. Sufferers often feel a burning inside the mouth and are more prone to developing mouth ulcers and infections, especially thrush. There are no particularly effective orthodox treatments. There is limited evidence to suggest that acupuncture can help; this may work more by giving patients relief rather than increasing the flow of saliva.[3]

Likelihood of being helped by acupuncture ●●

Nausea and vomiting
This is a common and distressing side-effect of many anti-cancer (chemotherapy) drugs. There are a number of medications that can effectively reduce these symptoms. Acupuncture can also help some people, but is more likely to relieve the vomiting than to reduce the nausea. Vomiting is most likely to be relieved with electro-acupuncture.[4]

Likelihood of being helped by acupuncture ●●●

Hot flushes
Women having treatment for breast cancer may experience early menopausal symptoms and distressing hot flushes. Acupuncture is definitely worth considering as orthodox HRT should not be used in women who have had breast cancer. My impression is that some women are definitely helped by acupuncture whilst others do not respond.[5]

Likelihood of being helped by acupuncture ●●●

Breathlessness

The breathlessness associated with cancer appears to be particularly amenable to acupuncture treatment.[6]

Likelihood of being helped by acupuncture ●●●

Notes to chapter 14

1 Paley CA et al. Acupuncture for cancer pain in adults. Cochrane Database Systematic Reviews 2011 Jan 19;(1):CD007753.

2 Molassiotis A et al. The management of cancer-related fatigue after chemotherapy with acupuncture and acupressure: a randomised controlled trial. Complementary Therapies in Medicine 2007; 15: 228-37.

3 O'Sullivan EM, Higginson IJ. Clinical effectiveness and safety of acupuncture in the treatment of irradiation-induced xerostomia in patients with head and neck cancer: a systematic review. Acupuncture in Medicine 2010; 28: 191-9.

4 Ezzo JM et al. Acupuncture-point stimulation for chemotherapy-induced nausea or vomiting. Cochrane Database of Systematic Reviews.(2):CD002285, 2006.

5 Lee MS et al. Acupuncture for treating hot flashes in breast cancer patients: a systematic review. Breast Cancer Res Treat 2009a; 115:497-503.

6 Filshie J, Penn K, Ashley S, Davis CL. Acupuncture for the relief of cancer-related breathlessness. Palliative Medicine. 1996;10(2):145-50.

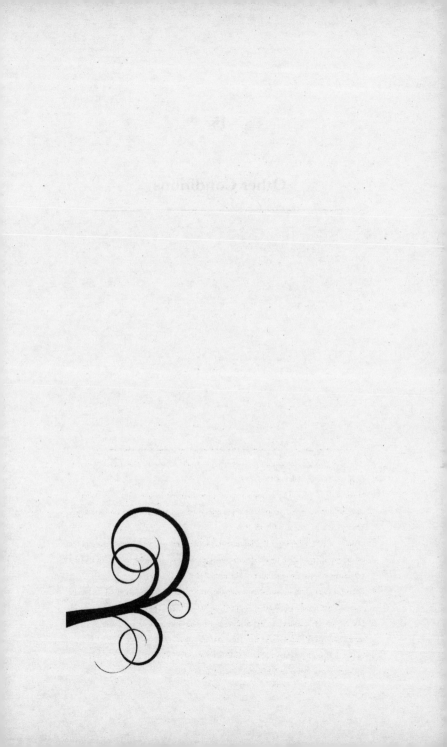

15

Other Conditions

Chronic or *recurrent cystitis* (also known as interstitial cystitis) is a common and distressing problem, mainly affecting women. It can result in the need to pass water urgently, frequently and often painfully. It can also make the sufferer have to get up at night several times to visit the bathroom. At its worst it can cause urinary incontinence. Drugs, and sometimes surgery, are used to treat the condition, but often not very successfully.

There is little research into acupuncture's effect on cystitis, but there is evidence that acupuncture may be very helpful in relieving the symptoms of this distressing condition.[1] Acupuncture appears to be just as effective as one of the most common drug treatments for this condition but with less side-effects.[2]

In a study of Norwegian women with recurrent urinary infections, three quarters of women were free from any urinary infection in the six months following a four-week course of acupuncture treatment, compared to half of the women who did not receive acupuncture.[3]

A course of 1-2 treatments a week for 4-6 weeks should be sufficient to judge whether acupuncture is likely to help any one individual.

Likelihood of being helped by acupuncture ●●●●

High blood pressure (hypertension) is extremely common, affecting one in three of the adult population, and usually requires lifelong treatment with medication. Acupuncture can reduce blood pressure – by an average of 10mm of mercury pressure – in hypertensive patients.[4,5]

This is similar to the effects of many of the most commonly used drugs to treat hypertension. Treatment may be needed at least twice weekly and the beneficial effect does not persist once acupuncture is stopped. So, like medication, treatment may need to be long-term.

Likelihood of being helped by acupuncture ●●

There is more evidence for the effectiveness of acupuncture in treating *nausea* and *vomiting* than for any other condition. Its use in 'early morning sickness' is discussed in Chapter 8 and its use in treating the nausea and vomiting associated with chemotherapy (for which electro-acupuncture may be particularly effective) in Chapter 13. It can also help relieve post-operative nausea and vomiting following surgery. For those with a dislike of needles, there is some good news as acupressure on its own also appears to be effective.[6]

Likelihood of being helped by acupuncture ●●●●●

Suffering a *stroke* is a devastating experience that often leaves the sufferer severely disabled. Unfortunately, strokes are common, affecting 150,000 people every year in the UK. A stroke is caused by a loss of blood supply to part of the brain, either because of a bleed (haemorrhage) or clot (thrombosis). This commonly results in permanent weakness in an arm or leg or down one side of the whole body. However many other problems can occur such as impaired speech or vision, confusion, unsteadiness and problems going to the toilet to urinate or defaecate.

Clearly anything extra that can aid recovery is to be welcomed.

There is good evidence that acupuncture is effective as an additional treatment alongside physical therapy. However acupuncture should not be used as an alternative to medical treatment, especially in the immediate aftermath of a stroke when early treatment may reduce the impact of the stroke. Acupuncture may be particularly effective in assisting recovery from stroke in those who are moderately to severely affected.[7,8]

There has been much debate about how much of the apparent beneficial effect of acupuncture in stroke recovery might be due to placebo, or the increased expectation the victim has that the acupuncture will aid recovery. This is partly because some studies seem to show that 'true' acupuncture (putting the needles in the 'right' place) is no more effective than 'sham' acupuncture (putting needles somewhere they are thought to have no effect). But as we are not certain where the best places to insert the needles are anyway, it is quite possible that the supposedly inactive 'sham' acupuncture may have some real effect.

In practice acupuncture is widely used in Eastern Europe (as well as, of course, China and Eastern Asia) for stroke patients.

Acupuncture is sometimes given as electro-acupuncture when used to aid recovery from stroke, and this is the method I personally prefer. Treatments should be given at least weekly, certainly in the early stages.

Likelihood of being helped by acupuncture ●●

Tinnitus is a condition causing a noise – often described as a buzzing or ringing – in one or both ears which, though often mild, can be extremely distressing. Nearly all of us have experienced it in the short term, for example following exposure to loud noise and as many as 1 in 10 have it all the time. Treatments range from counseling and relaxation therapy to white noise generators (devices that produce their own sound to distract from the tinnitus). Sadly acupuncture is unlikely to help most sufferers but may be a useful treatment in some individual patients.

Likelihood of being helped by acupuncture ○

In about half of the couples who are unable to conceive, *male infertility* (or subfertility) is the reason. There are many reasons for male infertility but one of the more common causes is a deficiency in the number or quality of sperm.

Several studies have demonstrated an increase in the quality and quantity of sperm following a course of acupuncture treatment.[9,10,11]

A raised temperature of the testes in the scrotum may be an important cause of male subfertility. Acupuncture treatment can reduce raised scrotal temperatures to normal levels and so may be a particularly effective treatment for men with infertility associated with raised scrotal temperatures.[12]

Likelihood of being helped by acupuncture ●●

Acupuncture is used for a variety of *skin conditions*. It would appear to have the potential to influence skin disease in several ways: it may have a local effect on the disease process or a general effect on the immune response; it may also relieve symptoms such as itch.

Acupuncture has been used for centuries in China to treat numerous skin conditions including acne, alopecia, dermatitis, pruritus (itching), psoriasis, rosacea, systemic lupus erythematosus (SLE) and urticaria (*See chapter 10*).[13] However, there is hardly any scientific research on the use of acupuncture to treat skin conditions and so difficult to come to any meaningful conclusions.

Likelihood of being helped by acupuncture ○

Research from China claims that acupuncture (and moxibustion) is safe and effective and may be better than western treatment of *acne.*[14]

Likelihood of being helped by acupuncture o

Shingles is caused by reactivation of the varicella-zoster virus that causes chickenpox. It is a common condition affecting 1 in 5 of us, usually in later life. After recovering from chickenpox the virus remains indefinitely – and usually harmlessly – in nerve endings in the spinal cord. At any stage in the future, sometimes triggered by stress or illness, the virus travels to the skin where it causes a few days of pain followed by the appearance of a localized blistering rash that can occur anywhere on the body. The big problem with shingles is that in one quarter of sufferers the pain (which is then called postherpetic neuralgia) persists after the rash has gone, sometimes for many months. There is no really satisfactory treatment for this pain which can be excruciatingly uncomfortable. Though there has been no research on this in the West, an overview from China concludes that acupuncture may help shorten the duration of shingles and, importantly, relieve the pain, possibly more effectively than commonly used Western medication.[15]

Likelihood of being helped by acupuncture ●●

Bell's Palsy is a one-sided weakness, or paralysis, of the face that comes on suddenly with no obvious cause. The condition improves on its own without treatment and most sufferers start to recover within a few weeks and three quarters make a full recovery, though this may take several months. 1 in 4 will be left with some degree of permanent facial weakness. Steroid tablets are often given to speed up recovery and they may also increase the chances of a full recovery.

Bell's Palsy is particularly common in China where acupuncture is used as a standard treatment for the condition. Acupuncture may also hasten recovery and increase the likelihood of a full recovery, possibly more effectively than steroids. Two or three treatments a week may be needed for maximum benefit.[16]

Likelihood of being helped by acupuncture ●●

Chronic Fatigue Syndrome (CFS) / Myalgic Encephalomyelitis (ME) is a disabling condition that causes severe tiredness which persists despite rest. People are affected most commonly in their 40s and 50s. The cause is unknown although it is sometimes precipitated by an infection, stress, an accident or possibly immunisation.

There is no satisfactory treatment; talking therapies such as Cognitive Behavioural Therapy (CBT) and medicines to treat symptoms are used. However, despite treatment, only one in 20 sufferers is able to return to normal functioning. It is not surprising that many turn to complementary therapies in order to try to get better. There have been several studies suggesting that acupuncture can help relieve physical and mental fatigue and improve the quality of life of patients with chronic fatigue syndrome. However, these results have been criticised for being of poor quality. Considering the poor recovery rate and the lack of alternative treatments it seems reasonable to try a course of acupuncture, perhaps six weekly treatments, to see if this can help to relieve symptoms.[17] A word of caution: sufferers of CFS/ME are often more susceptible to a temporary worsening of symptoms following treatment and so treatment should be very gentle initially.

Likelihood of being helped by acupuncture ○

Chronic Obstructive Pulmonary Disease COPD, which includes chronic bronchitis and emphysema, is a common cause of breathlessness mainly affecting older men and women who are smokers or ex-smokers. There is no cure but symptoms can be helped with inhalers ('puffers') and other medications. Those suffering severe symptoms require oxygen therapy.

There is a small amount of evidence to suggest that acupuncture can help relieve the distressing breathlessness associated with COPD. It appears less likely to objectively improve lung function but severe breathlessness is extremely upsetting and sufferers may be grateful for any relief they can obtain. Treatment may have to be long-term to maintain the subjective benefit.[18]

Likelihood of being helped by acupuncture ●●

Chronic, or *persistent*, *pain* is a huge problem affecting eight million people in the UK. Relentless pain can easily lead to depression and loss of work. Conditions that can cause persistent pain include arthritis, low back pain, headache and neuralgia and some of these are discussed in other chapters. Acupuncture is certainly good at relieving many types of pain so there is every reason to think that it can help relieve chronic pain.

The evidence does supports this to a degree. A thorough overview of all the evidence concluded that acupuncture does seem to be effective in relieving chronic pain compared to no treatment. However, as is so often the case with acupuncture research, real acupuncture did not appear to be convincingly superior to 'sham' or supposedly inactive acupuncture. I use the word 'supposedly' because it highlights a perennial problem with acupuncture research. The sceptics (and I have no objection to sceptics; I describe myself as an open-minded sceptic) argue that, in real scientific terms, acupuncture cannot be said to be truly effective until it can be demonstrated to be better than 'sham' or 'placebo' acupuncture.

However, sham acupuncture does usually involve inserting needles, but in different places to those traditionally thought to be correct and sometimes not deeply enough to be considered to be effective. The problem with this is that there is good evidence that inserting a needle anywhere in the body can have a real and significant effect on the body, affecting the nervous system, the brain and neuro-chemicals.

A more recent meta-analysis concluded that acupuncture had a real effect on alleviating chronic pain which was over and above any placebo effect. From a practical perspective acupuncture is certainly worth trying for chronic pain, particularly if other treatments are not working or causing troubling side-effects. At least six treatments may be necessary for the positive benefit of acupuncture to be felt.[19]

Likelihood of being helped by acupuncture ●●●

Diabetes is a common lifelong health condition affecting nearly three million people in the UK. Diabetes is the result of the sugar level in the blood being too high because of too little, or poorly functioning, insulin in the body. Around 1 in 10 diabetics have type 1 diabetes where the body is unable to produce any insulin. Type 1 diabetes is treated with daily injections of insulin. Type 2 diabetes occurs when the insulin produced by the body no longer works properly (called insulin resistance). It is much more common in older people. The treatment is often no more than eating a healthy diet and taking more exercise, though tablets, and even insulin injections, are needed by some. Diabetes affects nearly every part of the body and so there are many related problems or 'complications' that can occur. These include visual disturbances, kidney impairment, nerve damage causing lack of sensation and pain, and heart disease.

Acupuncture cannot replace orthodox treatment in diabetes and on no account should insulin be stopped if a diabetic receives acupuncture treatment.

Acupuncture is most likely to be helpful in diabetics suffering from *peripheral neuropathy*. This occurs as a result of nerve damage associated with diabetes. Common symptoms include numbness, tingling, pain and loss of sensation in the feet, legs, hands and arms. It can also cause problems with urination and digestion and erectile dysfunction in men. There is evidence that acupuncture can help relieve the pain of diabetic neuropathy. A course of six treatments given weekly should be sufficient to gauge whether acupuncture is likely to help or not.[20,21] Acupuncture may also help symptoms of *chronic cystitis/irritative bladder* (see page 115).

Likelihood of being helped by acupuncture ○ (for diabetes in general)

Likelihood of being helped by acupuncture ●● (for peripheral neuropathy)

Likelihood of being helped by acupuncture ●●●● (for irritative bladder)

Vertigo is the extremely unpleasant and disconcerting sensation of the world spinning round while you remain stationary. Anyone suffering from this should see their doctor as there are many causes requiring different treatments. In Menière's disease intermittent vertigo is accompanied by hearing loss and tinnitus (ringing in the ears – see page 119). It usually affects older people. There is no really satisfactory conventional treatment. There is some evidence that acupuncture can help relieve the vertigo of Menière's disease.[22]

Likelihood of being helped by acupuncture ○

Upper respiratory infections (the 'common cold') are the most common illnesses known to man. *Colds*, and *flu*, are caused by viruses and few of us get through a year without one. An enormous amount of money, time and effort has been invested in researching a cure for the common cold which, so far, has eluded us. Any treatment which shortened the length of colds, even by a day or two, would have an enormous impact on society because of the frequency of these infections. The best one can say is that acupuncture may help relieve some people of the symptoms of colds and flu.[23] Liz was seeing me for help with conception. She arrived one day with a blocked nose and headache as a result of a cold from which she was suffering. I offered to treat additional acupuncture points to try to relieve her cold symptoms. Having walked into my treatment room with a bad headache she left headache free and her remaining symptoms cleared up over the next couple of days. Acupuncture certainly seemed to have an effect on Liz's cold related headache.

Likelihood of being helped by acupuncture o

There is no evidence that acupuncture can cure *HIV* or *AIDS*. However it may help support the immune system and so help indirectly.

It is more likely that acupuncture has a role in treating some of the side-effects of the drug (anti-retroviral) therapy that is used to treat HIV. This commonly causes nausea, vomiting and headaches, which can be relieved with acupuncture.

Likelihood of being helped by acupuncture ○ (HIV itself)

Likelihood of being helped by acupuncture ●●● (nausea, vomiting and headaches of anti-retroviral treatment)

Cosmetic acupuncture, also known as facial rejuvenation acupuncture or 'acupuncture facelift' has become popular in recent years, not least because of its enthusiastic use by several celebrities. Fine acupuncture needles are inserted in the face and left in for 15 to 45 minutes. Treatments are often accompanied by a facial massage. Practitioners claim that facial acupuncture works primarily by increasing collagen production, though I can find no evidence for this, and that it also tones the muscles and tightens the skin. Most practitioners advise that at least 6, and up to 12, treatments are required in order to notice an improvement to your skin and then regular top-ups, every month or two, are often recommended.

Many acupuncture treatments involve inserting needles into the face, but cosmetic acupuncture itself appears to be a relatively new treatment, despite claims that it was popular with wealthy Chinese as long as one thousand years ago.

I remain sceptical about the effectiveness of cosmetic acupuncture but, provided it is given by an appropriately trained acupuncturist, should do no harm and is likely to be significantly cheaper and safer than surgery.

Likelihood of being helped by acupuncture ○

1 Aune A, Alraek T, LiHua H, Baerheim A. Acupuncture in the prophylaxis of recurrent lower urinary tract infection in adult women. Scandinavian Journal of Primary health Care 1998; 16(1): 37-39.

2 Kelleher CJ, Filshie J, Burton G, Khullar V, Cardozo LD. Acupuncture and the treatment of Irritative bladder symptoms. Acupuncture in Medicine 1994; 12(1): 9-12.

3 Alraek T, Soedal LIF, Fagerheim SU, Digranes A, Baerheim A. Acupuncture Treatment in the Prevention of Uncomplicated Recurrent Lower Urinary Tract Infections in Adult Women. American Journal of Public Health 2002; 92(10): 1609–1611.

4 Yin C, Seo B, Park H-J, Cho M, Jung W, et al. Acupuncture, a promising adjunctive therapy for essential hypertension: a double-blind randomized, controlled trial. Neurological Research 2007; 29 Suppl 1: S98-103.

5 Flachskampf FA, Gallasch J, Gefeller O, Gan J et al. Randomized trial of acupuncture to lower blood pressure. Circulation 2007; 115: 3121-9.

6 Ezzo J et al. Acupuncture-point stimulation for chemotherapy-induced nausea or vomiting. Cochrane Database of Systematic Reviews 2006b, Issue 2. Art. No.: CD002285. DOI: 10.1002/14651858.CD002285.pub2.

7 Shifflett SC, Samuel C. Does acupuncture work for stroke rehabilitation: what do recent clinical trials really show? Topics in Stroke Rehabilitation 2007; 14(4): 40-58.

8 Sällström S, Kjendahl A, Østen PE, Stanghelle JH, Borchgrevink CF. Acupuncture in the treatment of stroke patients in the subacute stage: a randomized controlled study. Complementary Therapies in Medicine 1996; 4: 193-197.

9 Siterman S, Eltes F, Wolfson V, Lederman H, Bartoov B. Does acupuncture treatment affect sperm density in males with very low sperm count? A pilot study. Andrologia 2000; 32: 31-39.

10 Gurfinkel E, Cedenho AP, Yamamura Y, Srougi M. Effects of acupuncture and moxa treatment in patients with semen abnormalities. Asian Journal of Andology 2003; 5(4): 345-8.

11 Siterman S, Eltes F, Wolfson V, Zabludovsky N, Bartoov B. Effect of acupuncture on sperm parameters of males suffering from subfertility related to low sperm quality. Archives of Andrology 1997; 39(2): 155-61.

12 Siterman S, Eltes F, Schechter L, Maimon Y, Lederman H, Bartoov B. Success of acupuncture treatment in patients with initially low sperm output is associated with a decrease in scrotal skin temperature. Asian Journal of Andrology 2009; 11(2): 200-8.

13 Tan EK, Millington GW, Levell NJ. Acupuncture in dermatology: an historical perspective. International Journal of Dermatology 2009; 48(6): 648-52.

14 Li B et al. Evaluation of therapeutic effect and safety for clinical randomized and controlled trials of treatment of acne with acupuncture and moxibustion. Zhongguo Zhenjiu [Chinese] 2009; 29: 247-51.

15 Yu XM et al. Systematic assessment of acupuncture for treatment of herpes zoster in domestic clinical studies. Zhongguo zhen jiu 2007; 27: 536-40.

16 Tong FM, Chow SK, Chan PY, Wong AK, Wan SS, Ng RK, Chan G, Chan WS, Ng A, Law CK . A prospective randomised controlled study on efficacies of acupuncture and steroid in treatment of idiopathic peripheral facial paralysis. Acupuncture in Medicine 2009 Dec; 27(4):169-73.

17 Wang T et al. A systematic review of acupuncture and moxibustion treatment for chronic fatigue syndrome in China. American Journal of Chinese Medicine 2008; 36:1-24.

18 Bausewein C et al. Non-pharmacological interventions for breathlessness in advanced stages of malignant and non-malignant diseases. Cochrane Database of Systematic Reviews 2008, Issue 2. Art. No.: CD005623. DOI: 10.1002/14651858.CD005623.pub2.

19 Vickers AJ et al. Acupuncture for chronic pain: individual patient data meta-analysis. Archives of Internal Medicine 2012; 172(19): 1444-53

20 Jiang H et al. Clinical study on the wrist-ankle acupuncture treatment for 30 cases of diabetic peripheral neuritis. J Tradit Chin Med. 2006 Mar;26(1):8-12.

21 Abuaisha BB et al. Acupuncture for the treatment of chronic painful peripheral diabetic neuropathy: a long-term study. Diabetes Res Clin Pract. 1998 Feb;39(2):115-21.

22 Long AF et al. Exploring the Evidence Base for Acupuncture in the Treatment of Meniere's Syndrome—A Systematic Review. Evidence-Based Complementary and Alternative Medicine 2011; doi:10.1093/ecam/nep047.

23 Kawakita K et al. Preventive and curative effects of acupuncture on the common cold: a multicentre randomized controlled trial in Japan. Complementary Therapies in Medicine 2004 Dec; 12: 181-8.

16

What Is Acupuncture Unable to Treat?

I have listed the conditions for which there is most scientific evidence that acupuncture can help and those that I personally feel are most likely to be helped by acupuncture.

Whilst most conditions not mentioned in this book are, in my view, less likely to be helped by acupuncture there may be exceptions in individual cases. The aim of any practitioner should be to try to find the right treatment for a particular individual with their specific problem. This is what I always tried to do as a GP, but is less likely to happen when you go to see a specialist.

If you visit an acupuncturist with a specific problem you are likely to receive acupuncture in the same way that if you visit a chiropractor you are likely to receive a manipulation and you will almost certainly he given a homoeopathic remedy after consultation with a homoeopath. The same applies to mainstream medicine where a referral to a surgeon is more likely to result in surgery than if you are referred to a physician. This is not surprising; after all, we all do what we do, and will offer help in what we are trained in.

What is most important when visiting an acupuncturist is that this does not prevent you from receiving treatment that might be more appropriate or even potentially life-saving. If you have cancer, by all means see an acupuncturist for help controlling symptoms but do not expect acupuncture to cure you. It is essential that you also see an orthodox specialist to receive, or at least be offered, treatment that is likely to be more appropriate. It may be stating the obvious when I say that a fracture needs to be treated in the fracture clinic, but then again acupuncture could have a role in supporting the healing process once the orthopaedic surgeons have fixed the initial break.

It is also important that patients seeking acupuncture for help with a specific condition do not stop taking their conventional medication unless this is agreed by their regular doctor. This particularly applies to conditions such as asthma, hypertension (high blood pressure), diabetes and thyroid disease in which long-term medication is needed to maintain health.

The bottom line is that acupuncture will of course not help everybody with every condition. For some conditions such as back pain, neck pain and nausea it will provide relief to most people receiving treatment.

For many other conditions only a minority will be helped but it is usually very difficult to tell who this minority will be.

Some people are not helped by acupuncture at all – for anything – while others appear to be particularly amenable to the benefits that acupuncture has to offer. In many cases the best course of action is to have a trial of a course of acupuncture to see whether it can help your particular problem; if there is no improvement after half a dozen treatments then it is unlikely that it is going to help.

Appendices

I

How Do I Find a Good Acupuncturist?

If you are very lucky you will have a GP or another doctor in your surgery who practices acupuncture. Failing that your local NHS physiotherapy unit may have a physiotherapist who uses acupuncture, though he or she may only treat muscular problems. Finally, if your problem is a longstanding painful one, you will find that acupuncture is offered in the vast majority of NHS pain clinics.

However, more often than not you will probably be unable to find acupuncture on the NHS and will then have no option but to find an acupuncturist in the 'Wild West' of the private sector. What follows is some guidance on how to find a private acupuncturist who is both competent and safe.

Anyone can, quite legally, set himself or herself up as an acupuncturist without any knowledge or training whatsoever. There is no statutory regulation of acupuncturists and so it is important to know how to find one who is safe and competent and you can trust to stick needles in you. The two most established organisations that cover the majority of acupuncturists practicing in the UK are the British Medical Acupuncture Society (BMAS) and the British Acupuncture Council (BAcC).

Western medical or Traditional Chinese acupuncture?

It is a little arbitrary to divide acupuncture treatment into two main types, especially as they overlap and some acupuncturists incorporate both systems into their practice. However, most acupuncturists do practice predominantly one form or the other and so it may be helpful to know which conditions are most likely to be helped by each method.

Western medical acupuncture, concentrating on trigger points is, in my experience, most effective for any muscular problems, as well as headaches, migraines and repetitive strain injuries (including tennis elbow). It can also be useful for conditions affecting the organs of the body (such as period pains, irritable bowel syndrome, colitis or chronic cystitis) when segmental acupuncture can be usefully employed (*See chapter 1*).

Traditional Chinese acupuncture is most helpful when people have symptoms that don't fit a traditional Western diagnosis such as feeling tired all the time or feeling generally unwell (provided causes treatable with conventional medicine have been excluded). TCM acupuncture is also more likely to be the first choice for conditions that affect much of the body, such as menopausal problems or PMS, and for conditions where acupuncture has been shown to be effective using Chinese methods such as nausea, vomiting and infertility.

It is generally a good idea to get a diagnosis from your own doctor first before visiting an acupuncturist to ensure that there isn't another treatment that would be more appropriate. It is probably safest to go to an acupuncturist who is a member of one of the following organisations.

The British Medical Acupuncture Society (BMAS)

The BMAS promotes Western scientific acupuncture. Its 2,700 members are all health professionals who are already regulated under their own regulatory body; these include doctors, physiotherapists, osteopaths, chiropractors and nurses. The BMAS runs training courses and educational events. Most BMAS members will be practicing acupuncture alongside more conventional techniques. Members are subject to its code of practice and complaints procedure.

There are several levels of membership of the BMAS:

Certificate of Basic Competence (CoBC):
The practitioner will have completed a BMAS Foundation Course or equivalent, practiced acupuncture for at least three months, keeping a logbook of over 30 cases, and demonstrated competence and safe practice to an experienced BMAS assessor.

Diploma in Western Medical Acupuncture (DipMedAc):
The practitioner will have completed the BMAS CoBC or SCA (see below), including the BMAS Foundation Course or equivalent. In addition, at least 100 training hours will have been completed including attending further courses and meetings, plus a logbook of at least 100 cases plus 15 detailed case reports. This level of training award is recognised by the BMAS for 'accredited' status, with reaccreditation required every five years by submission of a comprehensive training record comprising a minimum of 30 hours of further continuing professional development (CPD).

CPD is something that all health professionals should undertake. It is the way we continue to learn and develop throughout our careers in order to keep our skills and knowledge up to date and to work safely and effectively. Accredited members of the BMAS are likely to be recognised by health insurance providers such as BUPA and AXA PPP.

University of Hertfordshire qualifications

The BMAS now works with the University of Hertfordshire to offer a variety of qualifications ranging from a *safety and competence award (SCA)* through to an *MSc in Western Medical Acupuncture.*

However, it is important to bear in mind that all members of the BMAS are fully qualified health professionals in their own right in addition to practicing acupuncture.

British Acupuncture Council (BAcC)

The BAcC represents around 3,000 professional acupuncturists, most of whom practice traditional (Chinese) acupuncture.

All members are bound by the Council's codes of safe practice and professional conduct. Though the BAcC does not run its own training courses it accredits courses run by other organisations including several Universities.

Acupuncturists registered with the BAcC will have undertaken extensive training in traditional Chinese medicine and acupuncture along with training in anatomy, physiology and pathology, amounting to a total of 3,600 hours of study. They are also required to undertake CPD.

Acupuncture Association of Chartered Physiotherapists (AACP)

The AACP has over 6,000 physiotherapist members who have undertaken at least 80 hours of training on acupuncture. An advanced member will have a minimum of 200 hours of acupuncture training. All members are required to undertake at least ten hours of acupuncture training every two years. AACP acupuncturists may be most appropriate for muscular problems.

British Academy of Western Medical Acupuncture (BAWMA)

The BAWMA has run acupuncture courses, with an emphasis on Western scientific acupuncture, for many doctors, nurses and physiotherapists during the last 30 years or so that it has existed. It has around 1,500 members, most of whom work in the NHS, and are required to undertake annual CPD.

The Acupuncture Society

The Acupuncture Society represents around 600 practitioners of Chinese and Oriental medicine including acupuncture, Chinese herbal medicine, acupressure and Tui na (a type of massage therapy). Members are subject to the Society's code of ethics, rules and regulation and must undertake 15 hours of CPD a year (shortly to be increased to 30 hours a year).

If you have any doubts about the competence of your acupuncturist you should ask the following questions:

1. Where were you trained in acupuncture?

There are many places that offer good courses in acupuncture, both in the UK and abroad. It is important that the acupuncturist has had sufficient training particularly if he or she is not a health care professional with other qualifications. If you want to find out more about your acupuncturist's training then get in touch with the training establishment or the accrediting organisation (such as the BAcC or Acupuncture Society).

2. What qualifications do you have?

This is a bit of a minefield as there are so many qualifications from a large number of training bodies. Members of the BAcC will have MBAcC after their name. Doctors and other health professionals will have their own professional qualifications.

3. What experience do you have?

You could ask your acupuncturist how long he or she

has been practicing and how many patients he or she treats every week. In most fields of healthcare experience leads to better practice.

4. What sort of needles do you use?
Sterile single use disposable needles should always be used. Do not get treated by someone using reusable needles.

5. Do you have professional insurance?
All acupuncturists should have professional liability insurance.

A personal recommendation is also valuable. Try asking your GP if he or she is able to recommend a local acupuncturist. Perhaps a friend or colleague has had a good experience visiting an acupuncturist; this doesn't guarantee that the acupuncturist in question is competent and safe, but it is a good start. Also trust your instincts. It is essential you have confidence in someone who is about to stick needles into you.

How much does private acupuncture cost?

This will vary widely and depend on the practitioner's qualifications, experience and location.

Most practitioners have slightly longer initial appointments (lasting from 30 minutes up to an hour or more) so that they can take a full history and do any necessary examinations before giving you your first treatment. Subsequent appointments are likely to be shorter but the length will depend on the type of acupuncture practiced.

Costs are anything from £40 up to £100 or more for the initial consultation and treatment and from £35 to £100 for subsequent treatments.

Is acupuncture covered by private health insurance?

If you are fortunate enough to have private health insurance, most policies will include a provision for acupuncture, though the amount of cover varies widely from policy to policy, so you will have to contact your insurer to find out exactly what cover your policy offers.

However not all acupuncturists will be recognised by private health insurance, though the criteria will vary from insurer to insurer. For example, at the time of writing, BUPA will only cover medically qualified acupuncturists who hold the higher (Dip Med Ac) BMAS qualification. On the other hand AXA PPP also recognises acupuncturists registered with the BAcC.

Donating blood after acupuncture

In some circumstances you may not be allowed to

donate blood for a period after receiving acupuncture. The guidelines in England and Wales are that if you have received acupuncture you should wait for four months before giving blood. This is because of the risk of infection if the acupuncture was performed using non-sterile needles or with a bad technique.

However, if your acupuncture was performed by NHS staff on NHS premises or was performed outside the NHS but by a qualified Health Care Professional, registered with a statutory body, such as a doctor or physiotherapist, then you may donate immediately.

If you have had acupuncture outside the NHS and this was not performed by a qualified Health Care Professional registered with a statutory body, then you are asked to wait four months from your last treatment before donating. This applies to acupuncturists who are members of the BAcC as this is a non statutory body. If your treatment was between 4 and 12 months ago, you must disclose this when you give blood as you will need an additional blood test prior to giving blood.

II

Research into Acupuncture

There is considerable ongoing research into acupuncture but this still remains far less than research on medical drugs which is largely funded by the wealthy pharmaceutical companies. However, there are numerous difficulties associated with scientific research into acupuncture.

Much of the research has been done in China. Not only does this mean that it is written in Chinese, but also much of this research lacks the scientific rigour that is demanded by scientists in the West. For example, it is common for studies not to have 'controls', that is a group of patients with the same condition who were not treated with acupuncture, or treated with something different, with whom to compare the treated patients. It is of course very rewarding if patients given acupuncture get better. However, if patients not receiving acupuncture improve just as much then acupuncture is offering no additional benefit. It is for this reason that it is considered very important to have a 'control' group of patients with whom the treated group can be compared.

Placebo

Another criticism of acupuncture is that it is merely 'placebo' or that any beneficial effect happens simply because the patient believes in acupuncture or it would have happened anyway without treatment. The argument goes that patients treated with acupuncture may improve more than patients on no treatment but that this is purely due to the powerful psychological effect of having needles inserted accompanied by the patients' belief that acupuncture will work. For this reason 'real' acupuncture is often compared to pretend or 'sham' acupuncture. In order for this 'sham' acupuncture to be a true placebo it must be indistinguishable to the patient from real acupuncture but have no real effect. Placebo 'sham' acupuncture can take many different forms. One way that has often been used is to insert acupuncture needles in places where they are not expected to have any clinical effect. However it is now thought that inserting needles anywhere in the body may produce a positive benefit; if this is the case then it cannot be used as an inert comparison to 'real' acupuncture.

In order to try and get round this problem a fake acupuncture needle has been devised that works rather like a theatrical dagger. When inserted it appears to go into the skin but actually retreats into its holding case. This has shown to be a reasonably effective 'placebo' in that patients often think that they are having a needle inserted into their skin, i.e. real acupuncture. However it has been argued that even these could exert some clinical effect as they do actually touch, and therefore stimulate, the skin even though the skin is not penetrated. Indeed studies have shown that merely touching the skin with the blunt end of a needle can have profound effects on areas of the brain.

So the problem of what to use as 'sham' or 'placebo' acupuncture remains unsolved. Thankfully this does not prevent ongoing research from taking place.

The German insurance company trials

In the early 21st-century several German health insurance companies paid for a series of large studies looking at the effect of acupuncture on patients with various conditions. These companies had been reimbursing patients for acupuncture treatment but finding it increasingly expensive. In order to decide whether to continue reimbursing patients they ran a series of large studies looking at the effect of acupuncture on headache (tension headache or migraine), neck pain, back pain, and knee and hip osteoarthritis.

All the patients in the trials were randomly divided into one of three groups: some received real acupuncture, some received sham acupuncture involving insert-ing needles only a little way under the skin into points that would not, traditionally, be expected to have any clinical effect, and the remainder were put on a waiting list for acupuncture at a future date. At the end of the treatments patients who had received true acupuncture were more improved than those who had sham acupuncture in nearly all studies though often the dif-ferences were not great.

What was particularly interesting was that both the real acupuncture and sham acupuncture treated patients did much better those left on the waiting list for nearly all the conditions treated. Clearly patients benefited from acupuncture treatment, but this has led to a vigor-ous debate in the acupuncture community over whether it is important or not to needle at specific points or whether inserting needles virtually anywhere on the body will have the same positive effect. I have no doubt this debate will continue for many years to come.

What these large and well-designed trials did show is that:

1   acupuncture works just as well as best stan-dard medical care for migraine

2   acupuncture is much better than best standard medical care for both low back pain and osteoarthritis of the knee

3   real acupuncture appears to be more effective

than sham acupuncture (as performed in these trials) though the differences were much less than between both real and sham acupuncture and no treatment.

On the strength of these results the German insurance organisations decided to provide funding for acupuncture treatment of both osteoarthritis of the knee and back pain.

III

Resources

_____

The British Medical Acupuncture Society (BMAS)
All its members are statutorily registered health professionals who practice acupuncture. The society promotes evidence-based acupuncture and can provide details of acupuncturists with different levels of qualification in your area.
www.medical-acupuncture.co.uk
Tel: 01606 786782 or 020 7713 9437

The British Acupuncture Council (BAcC)
BAcC members mainly practice traditional Chinese acupuncture. The Council can put you in touch with members local to you.
www.acupuncture.org.uk
Tel: 020 8735 0400

Acupuncture Association of Chartered Physiotherapists (AACP)
The AACP can put you in touch with physiotherapists local to you who practice acupuncture.
www.aacp.org.uk

British Academy of Western Medical Acupuncture

(BAWMA)

BAWMA is based in the North-west of England. It has around 1,500 members, most of whom work in the NHS.

www.bawma.co.uk

The Acupuncture Society

The Acupuncture Society represents practitioners of Chinese acupuncture and other Chinese and Oriental therapies.

www.acupuncturesociety.org.uk

City Acupuncture

This is the author's acupuncture web site and includes information about acupuncture and what conditions acupuncture can best help. It also has information on his clinic situated at the Broadgate Spine and Joint Clinic in London.

www.cityacupuncture.org.uk

NHS Choices

Here you can find limited information on acupuncture. www.nhs.uk/Conditions/Acupuncture/Pages/Introduction.aspx

BUPA

The BUPA website also provides some information on acupuncture

http://www.bupa.co.uk/individuals/health-information/directory/a/acupuncture

Australia

In Australia acupuncture practice is in the process of becoming regulated. Currently regulation varies from state to state.

Australian Acupuncture & Chinese Medicine Association Ltd (AACMA)
The AACMA represent over 2,200 acupuncturists and Chinese medicine practitioners. AACMA acupuncturists are likely to use a traditional Chinese medical approach.
www.acupuncture.org.au

Acupuncture Association of Australia Inc.
All members are registered health practitioners, including doctors, nurses, physiotherapist, osteopaths and chiropractors, who have also completed relevant acupuncture qualifications.
www.acupaa.com.au

Federation of Chinese Medicine & Acupuncture Societies of Australia Ltd (FCMA)
The FCMA represents more than 700 practitioners. All members hold a minimum of a Chinese medicine bachelor degree or the equivalent and are bound by a code of ethics.
www.fcma.org.au

New Zealand

Acupuncture is currently not regulated in New Zealand.

New Zealand Register of Acupuncturists (NZRA)
The NZRA is the largest professional body represent-

ing practitioners of acupuncture and Chinese medicine in New Zealand. Members are bound by the NZRA rules and code of professional ethics. They will have completed the equivalent of four years full-time training and are required to complete ongoing professional education.

www.acupuncture.org.nz

New Zealand Acupuncture Standards Authority (NZASA)
The NZASA is a voluntary self-regulatory body that registers acupuncturists in New Zealand

www.nzasa.org

Physiotherapy Acupuncture Association of New Zealand Inc. (PAANZ)
PAANZ represent physiotherapists with a special interest in acupuncture. Members must have completed at least 80 jours of acupuncture training. Registered Physiotherapy Acupuncturists have obtained a minimum of 150 hours of PAANZ approved training and must undertake continuing training an professional development.

www.paanz.org.nz

Somer Further Reading

An Introduction to Western Medical Acupuncture. Edited by Adrian White, Mike Cummings & Jacqueline Filshie. Churchill Livingstone 2008.

The Web that has no Weaver by Ted Kaptchuk. Contemporary Books 2000.

Index

Acne 121
Acupressure 24-5
Addiction 88-9
AIDS 132
Alcohol addiction 90
Allergic conditions, other 86
Anxiety 101-2
Asthma 83-4

Back pain, low 41-2, 78
Bell's Palsy 123
Breech presentation 76

Cancer 106-110
Central regulatory effects 18-9
Chronic Fatigue Syndrome (CFS) 124
Chronic Obstructive Pulmonary Disease (COPD) 125
Cocaine addiction 90
Colds 131
Cosmetic acupuncture 25, 133
Cupping 25
Cystitis, chronic 113

Depression 103-4
Diabetes 128-9

Ear (auricular) acupuncture 23-4
Eating 91
Electro-acupuncture 21
Endometriosis 69
Extrasegmental acupuncture 18

Fibromyalgia 50
Flu 131
Frozen shoulder 51

Hay fever 85

Herpes zoster 122
High blood pressure 114
HIV 132
Hypertension 114

Infertility, male 119
Infertility, female 67-8
Inflammatory bowel disease 97-8
Insomnia 101-2
Irritable Bowel Syndrome (IBS) 95-6
Irritative bladder 113

Labour 79
Laser acupuncture 24
Local stimulation 17

Menière's disease 130
Menopausal symptoms 62-4
Migraine 56-7
Mild side-effects 32
Moxibustion 22
Muscular conditions, other 52
Myalgic Encephalomyelitis (ME) 124

Nausea 75, 108, 115
Neck pain 43
Needles 21

Opiate addiction 90
Osteoarthritis (OA) 44-5

Pain, chronic 126-7
Period pain 61
Polycystic Ovarian

Syndrome (PCOS) 65-6
Pregnancy, indigestion 77; labour 79; low back and pelvic pain 78; morning sickness 75
Premenstrual Syndrome (PMS) 70-1

Repetitive Strain Injury (RSI) 49
Rheumatoid arthritis (RA) 46
Reactions to acupuncture 32-3

Segmental acupuncture 17-8
Shingles 122
Skin conditions 120
Smoking, stoping 89
Stress 101-102
Stroke 116-117

Tennis elbow 47-8
Tension headache 55
Tinnitus 118
Traditional Chinese Medicine (TCM) 14-6, 142-3
Trigger point acupuncture 19, 22-3

Vertigo 130
Vomiting 75, 108, 115

Weight loss 91
Western Medical Acupuncture 16-9, 142-3